THE BOOK OF HEARTS

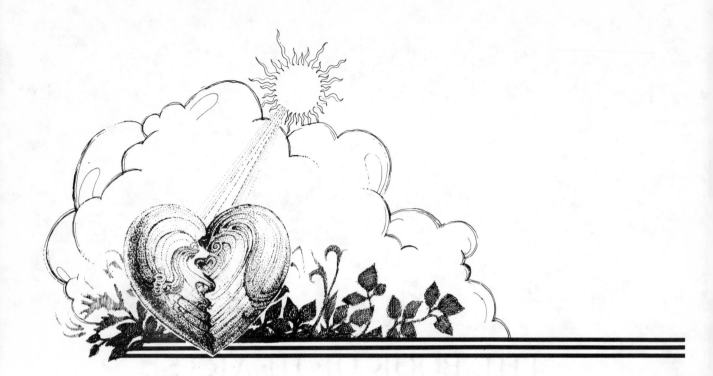

The BOOK of HEARTS

Edited by Peter John Dorman

Design by Claire Owen
Illustration by Michael Green

RUNNING PRESS
PHILADELPHIA, PENNSYLVANIA

Acknowledgments

Grateful acknowledgment is made to the following for permission to reproduce materials. In the listing below, titles preceded by an asterisk are not part of the original copyrighted material.

*A Hearty Dish from India, p. 11: From *Cooking of the Maharajas*, by S.R. and S.D. Holkar; ©1975 by The Viking Press. *The Walking Heart, p. 12: From "Walking," by Jack Galub, *Glamour*, June 1978; copyright ©1978 by The Conde Nast Publications, Inc. Heart-Burial, p. 14: Reprinted with permission from *Encyclopaedia Britannica*, 11th edition, ©1910-11 by Encyclopaedia Britannica, Inc. *Never Bet the Devil Your Heart, p. 16: From *The Enlarged Devil's Dictionary*, ©1967 by Ernest J. Hopkins; reprinted by permission of Doubleday & Company. *The Unabridged Heart, p. 17: Reprinted by permission from *Webster's Third New International Dictionary* © 1976 by G. & C. Merriam Co., Publishers of the Merriam-Webster Dictionaries. A Man All Heart, p. 22: From *A Dictionary of British Folk-Tales*, by Katharine M. Briggs; Part A, Folk Narratives, Vol. 2; copyright © 1970 by K.M. Briggs; reprinted by permission of Indiana University Press. *Reflections on Heart Transplants, p. 31: From *Biological Systems*, by Shelby D. Gerking; © 1974 by W.B. Saunders Company. *The Purest Theatre, p. 31; *The Bower of Love, p. 55; The Garrulous Heart, p. 69: From *Mortal Lessons*, copyright © 1974, 1975, 1976 by Richard Selzer; reprinted by permission of Simon & Schuster, a Division of Gulf & Western Corporation. *Cross My Heart, p. 47: Copyright © 1976 by The New York Times Company; reprinted by permission. *The Nutritious Heart, p. 51: Reprinted by permission from *Barbara Kraus Dictionary of Protein*, © 1975 by Harper & Row, Publishers, Inc. Pickled Venison Heart, p. 73; Pickled Elk's Heart, p. 89: Reprinted by permission of G.P. Putnam's Sons from *The New York Times Heritage Cook Book* by Jean Hewitt; copyright ©1972 by The New York Times. *Heartbroken, p. 93: Reprinted with permission from *Stedman's Medical Dictionary*, ©1961 by The Williams & Wilkins Company, Baltimore.

I would also like to thank Richard E. Nicholls and Alida Becker for their numerous editorial contributions; and Betty Holop for providing "Broadway Hearts," "With a Heart in My Song," and "Hearts of Gold." Special thanks go to Richard Scholl, Research Consultant, for uncovering many of the materials that eventually found their way into this book.

Canadian representatives: John Wiley & Sons, Ltd. 22 Worcester Road, Rexdale, Ontario M9W 1L1

International representatives: Kaiman & Polon, Inc. 2175 Lemoine Avenue, Fort Lee, New Jersey 07024

Digit on the right indicates the number of this printing.

9 8 7 6 5 4 3 2 1

Library of Congress Cataloging in Publication Data
The Book of Hearts.
    SUMMARY: Facts, myths, quotes, and other curiousa about the heart.
    1. Heart (in religion, folklore, etc.)   2. Heart—Miscellanea.
    [1. Heart (in religion, folklore, etc.)   2. Heart—Miscellanea.]
GR489.B6   398.2   78-14898
    I. Dorman, Peter J.
ISBN 0-89471-045-1 library binding
ISBN 0-89471-044-3 paperback

Cover illustration by Tony Mascio
Cover art direction by James Wizard Wilson

Typography: Paladium, with Tiffany, by Type & Stat House, Inc., Philadelphia, Pennsylvania
Printed and bound by Port City Press, Baltimore, Maryland

This book may be ordered directly from the publisher. Please include 25 cents postage.

TRY YOUR BOOKSTORE FIRST.

Running Press
38 South Nineteenth Street
Philadelphia, Pennsylvania 19103

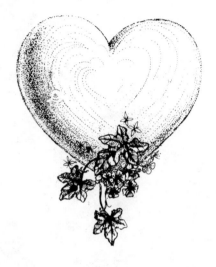

WHAT?   Publish a Heart?

"Perhaps," muses surgeon-poet Richard Selzer, "if one were to cut out a heart, a lobe of the liver, a single convolution of the brain, and paste it to a page, it would speak with more eloquence than all the words of Balzac. Such a piece would need no literary style, no mass of erudition or history, but in its very shape and feel would tell all the frailty and strength, the despair and nobility of man. What? Publish a heart? A little piece of bone? Preposterous. Still I fear that is what it may require to reveal the truth that lies hidden in the body."

Yes, in a sense the heart of man embodies his history. We make no pretense of covering that story. Instead, we invite you to share a glimpse of some of the eloquence, whimsy, and knowledge that have been inspired by the ten ounces of beating muscle which is the pulse of every human life.

What? Publish a heart and paste it to a page? No, we believe the printing process is a bit tidier. And surely *The Book of Hearts* will show you more of the myriad ways in which the human mind expresses its fascination with the human heart.

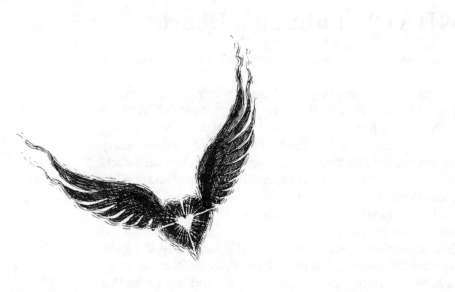

Heart-a-facts
Heart-a-facts

Sudden happiness increases the heart rate. So does sudden anger.

Bigger people have bigger hearts.

The human heart weighs about 1/200th of the total body weight.

The heart beats continuously from the fifth month before birth until death.

Each heartbeat lasts about eight-tenths of a second.

On the average, the human heart beats 72 times a minute, or about 100,000 times a day, or about 38,000,000 times a year.

The human heart beats about 4 billion times during an average lifetime.

In one minute, the heart pumps from 8 to ten pints of blood through 60,000 miles of blood vessels—that's more than twice around the world.

In one day, the heart pumps the equivalent of 5000 gallons of blood through the body.

Heart attack is a non-specific term that usually refers to a myo-cardial infarction.

Initially, an experience of fear lowers the heart rate.

The heart rate is at its highest in the early afternoon and at its lowest in the morning.

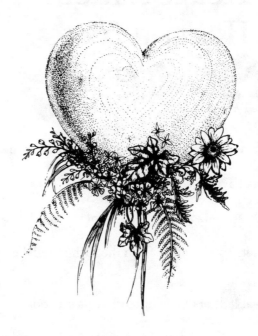

FOOD OF THE GODS

When the Aztecs spoke of the "food of the gods," they were referring to the human heart—and not in any symbolic way. Their gods were hungry gods, demanding a steady diet of hearts if they were to keep the universe in order.

The Aztec domination of central Mexico lasted only a little over a hundred years, ending when they were overthrown by Cortes and his conquistadores in the sixteenth century. But in that short span of time, the Aztecs may have sacrificed hundreds of thousands of people to their gods.

Every year, some fifteen thousand prisoners (most of them captured during the Aztecs' many wars and raids) were led up to the temples atop the great stone pyramids. There they were spreadeagled on a sacrificial stone and killed by the single stroke of an obsidian knife which tore the hearts from their bodies. The hearts were then ritually offered to the gods and cast into a brazier to be burned.

"Heart-string" has been defined as a hypothetical nerve or tendon, supposed to brace and sustain the heart.

10

A Hearty Dish from India

1 lb. heart (approximately 4-5
lamb hearts or 1 veal heart)

Two hours before serving, wash the hearts under cold running water; trim off any fatty covering and tubes, but leave the heart whole. Cover with cold water in a small saucepan and bring to rolling boil. Discard this water; rinse the hearts thoroughly and repeat this procedure once again.

1 cup unpeeled garlic cloves
1 tablespoon powdered cumin

Drop the garlic and cumin into the blender and add 1/2 cup water. Blend and scrape to a paste. Coat the blanched and rinsed hearts in this paste and leave thus unrefrigerated until they are to be cooked (minimum 1 hour).

2 tablespoons ground sweet fennel,
or 2 tablespoons whole fennel,
coarsely ground in blender

After they have marinated, rinse the hearts thoroughly. Cover with cold water in a small saucepan; add the fennel and again bring to a boil. Then reduce the heat and simmer uncovered for 10 minutes. Discard the water; rinse the hearts and slice as thinly as possible with a sharp knife.

Preheat oven to warm (200°F.)

1/3 cup clarified butter
2 cups onion, cut in half from top to root,
and across the grain into thin, even slices
1/2 teaspoon salt
1/2 teaspoon powdered cardamom

Heat the butter in a medium-sized casserole and fry the onions until brown but not crisp. Stir in the slices of heart, salt, and cardamom. Cover and leave in a warm oven for 15-20 minutes.

SERVES 2-3

"The way to the heart is through the senses; please the eyes and ears, and the work is half done."—Lord Chesterfield

"The poor human heart must break piecemeal."
—Georg Herwegh

"The thing that eats the heart," writes Stanley Kunitz, *"is mostly heart."*

The Walking Heart

"Most of us do not realize that even moderate slopes cause the heart to work harder, helping to raise the pulse rate to what we consider the target or training-effect zone," says Dr. Borisse Paulin. "If the heart is made to beat within this zone for a half-hour or more a day, its stamina increases. In fact, the total cardiovascular system becomes more efficient."

Your "target zone" is easy to compute: It is 70 to 75 percent of your maximum heartbeat. For a twenty-year-old, the maximum heart rate is 200 beats per minute, so the target zone would be 140-150 beats per minute. (For other maximums and target zones, see the table below. The maximum heart rate is 200 beats; for each year after twenty, the maximum decreases approximately one beat per minute.) An exercise or training pulse rate of 70 to 75 percent of your age-related maximum is comfortable and safe for most walkers who are in good health. Unless you are training for the Olympics, exercising vigorously enough to bring your heart rate up to near-maximum is unnecessary, and for most people impossible. It is a good idea to check with your doctor before beginning any vigorous exercise program.

The Greek physician Galen was born in the year 130 A.D. Today he is remembered primarily for his extensive theoretical writings on medicine and the human body. Much of Galen's knowledge of anatomy was gathered first-hand during the time he served as physician to the gladiators who performed in the city of Pergamon.

Galen treated many gladiators who had been wounded in the heart. While such injuries were invariably fatal, some of the men might linger on for as long as a day and a night. Galen wrote that these men retained their senses until the end, thus refuting the belief, passed down from the Sumerians, that the heart was the seat of man's intelligence.

AGE	MAXIMUM HEART RATE	70-75% TARGET ZONE
20	200	140-150
22	198	139-148
24	196	137-147
26	194	135-146
28	192	134-144
30	190	133-143
32	189	132-142
34	187	131-140
36	186	130-139

Pulse rates are easily determined. After walking briskly for at least five minutes, stop and immediately count your pulse at your wrist or side of your neck for ten seconds, then multiply by six.

"The heart is like the tree that gives balm for the wounds of man, only when the iron has wounded it."—Chateaubriand

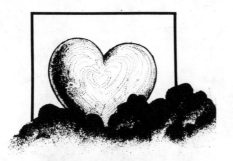

THE WORLD'S LARGEST VALENTINE

For over twenty years, the Franklin Institute has had the distinction of being the only cultural and educational institution in Philadelphia which actually has a heart. Built in 1953, the museum's famous walk-through model of a human heart is 28 feet wide and 18 feet high—almost 15,000 times larger than a human heart. Accompanied by a recording of the sounds of a beating heart, visitors travel the route a blood corpuscle takes as it pumps through the heart. Along the way, they can see and touch larger-than-life reproductions of the strategic parts of the organ.

To construct the giant heart, designers used cross sections of frozen beef hearts to produce drawings that were projected on plywood and cut out in concentric, interlocking rings. These were hooked together using 4,000 square feet of metal lath and 4 tons of papier mache. The exhibit was originally intended to be only a temporary structure, but from its unveiling it has drawn such crowds that it has never been dismantled. Now, 23 years and 10 million visitors later, the heart is in need of major surgery, and the Franklin Institute has launched a one-hundred-thousand-dollar heart rehabilitation program.

But O heart! heart! heart!
O the bleeding drops of red,
Where on the deck my Captain lies
Fallen cold and dead.
                    —Walt Whitman

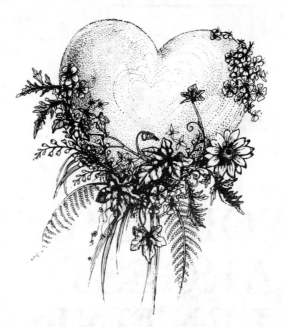

HEART-BURIAL

Heart-Burial is the burial of the heart apart from the body. This is a very ancient practice, the special reverence shown towards the heart being doubtless due to its early association with the soul of man, his affections, courage and conscience. In medieval Europe heart-burial was fairly common. Some of the more notable cases are those of Richard I., whose heart, preserved in a casket, was placed in Rouen cathedral; Henry III., buried in Normandy; Eleanor, queen of Edward I., at Lincoln; Edward I., at Jerusalem; Louis IX., Philip III., Louis XIII. and Louis XIV., in Paris. Since the 17th century the hearts of deceased members of the house of Hapsburg have been buried apart from the body in the Loretto chapel in the Augustiner Kirche, Vienna. The most romantic story of heart-burial is that of Robert Bruce. He wished his heart to rest at Jerusalem in the church of the Holy Sepulchre, and on his deathbed entrusted the fulfillment of his wish to Douglas. The latter broke his journey to join the Spaniards in their war with the Moorish king of Granada, and was killed in battle, the heart of Bruce enclosed in a silver casket hanging around his neck. Subsequently the heart was buried at Melrose Abbey. The heart of

"When Basutos (African tribe) of the mountains have killed a very brave foe, they immediately cut out his heart and eat it, because this is supposed to give them his courage and strength in battle. When Sir Charles M'Carthy was killed by the Ashantees in 1824, it is said that his heart was devoured by the chiefs of the Ashantee army, who hoped by this means to imbibe his courage."—*Sir George Frazer*

James, marquess of Montrose, executed by the Scottish Covenanters in 1650, was recovered from his body, which had been buried by the roadside outside Edinburgh, and, enclosed in a steel box, was sent to the duke of Montrose, then in exile. It was lost on its journey, and years afterwards was discovered in a curiosity shop in Flanders. Taken by a member of the Montrose family to India, it was stolen as an amulet by a native chief, was once more regained, and finally lost in France during the Revolution. Of notable 17th-century cases there is that of James II., whose heart was buried in the church of the convent of the Visitation at Chaillot near Paris, and that of Sir William Temple, at Moor Park, Farnham.

The last ceremonial burial of a heart in England was that of Paul Whitehead, secretary to the Monks of Medmenham club, in 1775, the interment taking place in the Le Despenser mausoleum at High Wycombe, Bucks. Of later cases the most notable are those of Daniel O'Connell, whose heart is at Rome, Shelley at Bournemouth, Louis XVII. at Venice, Kosciusko at the Polish museum at Rapperschwyll, Lake Zurich, and the marquess of Bute, taken by his widow to Jerusalem for burial in 1900. Sometimes other parts of the body, removed in the process of embalming, are given separate and solemn burial. Thus the viscera of the popes from Sixtus V. (1590) onward have been preserved in the parish church of the Quirinal. The custom of heart-burial was forbidden by Pope Boniface VIII. (1294-1303), but Benedict XI. withdrew the prohibition.

Bury My Heart in Missolonghi

Ostracized from English society after scandal and controversy, Lord Byron—once the charismatic darling of the English Romantics—gave his heart to the cause of Greek liberty. He died in 1824, consummating a period of fervent and whole-heartedly exhaustive efforts on behalf of Greece's revolution against the Turks. General mourning among the Greek populace continued for twenty-one days. When Byron's body was eventually carried back to England, his heart, at the request of the Greek government, remained in Greece. In the town of Missolonghi, the site of Byron's noblest actions, a small monument was raised to commemorate the heart that lay entombed beneath it.

The good die first,
And they whose hearts
*   are dry as summer dust*
Burn to the socket.
                    —William Wordsworth

"A good heart is worth gold."—Shakespeare

"All who know their own minds, do not know
their own hearts."—Rochefoucauld

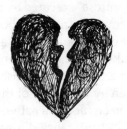

Never Bet
the Devil
Your Heart

A Definition, by Ambrose Bierce

HEART, *n.* An automatic muscular bloodpump. Figuratively, this useful organ is said to be the seat of emotions and sentiments—a very pretty fancy which, however, is nothing but a survival of a once universal belief. It is now known that the sentiments and emotions reside in the stomach, being evolved from food by chemical action of the gastric fluid. The exact process by which a beefsteak becomes a feeling—tender or not, according to the age of the animal from which it was cut; the successive stages of elaboration through which a caviar sandwich is transmuted to a quaint fancy and reappears as a pungent epigram; the marvelous functional methods of converting a hard-boiled egg into religious contrition, or a creampuff into a sigh of sensibility—these things have been patiently ascertained by M. Pasteur, and by him expounded with convincing lucidity. (See, also, my monograph, *The Essential Identity of the Spiritual Affections and Certain Intestinal Gases Freed in Digestion*—4to, 687 pp.) In a scientific work entitled, I believe, *Delectatio Demonorum* (John Camden Hotton, London, 1873) this view of the sentiments receives a striking illustration; and for further light consult Professor Dam's famous treatise on *Love as a Product of Alimentary Maceration.*

Some Offbeat Hearts

Heartburn: a bad cigar.
Heart's ease: a twenty-shilling piece.
Hearts: amphetamines.
Heart bag: a heart-shaped tobacco pouch.
Hearts of oak: penniless; broke.
Heartbreaker: a lovelock, a loose ringlet worn over the shoulders, or curl over the temples. Also, a flirt.

16

¹heart \'härt, 'hȧt, *usu* -d·+V\ *n* -s [ME *hert*, fr. OE *heorte*;

heart 1a, showing course of the blood coming from the body and entering from *1* superior vena cava and from *2* inferior vena cava; to *3* right atrium; to *4* right ventricle; to *5* pulmonary artery; to *6* lungs (not shown); to *7* pulmonary veins; to *8* left atrium; to *9* left ventricle; to *10* aorta; leaving by *11* to the head, neck, and upper extremities (not shown)

akin to OHG *herza* heart, ON *hjarta*, Goth *hairto*, L *cord-*, *cor*, OIr *cride*, Gk *kardia*, Arm *sirt*, Hitt *karts*] **1 a :** a hollow muscular organ of vertebrate animals that by its rhythmic contraction acts as a force pump maintaining the circulation of the blood, is in the human adult about five inches long and three and one half broad, of conical form, is placed obliquely in the chest with the broad end upward and to the right and the apex opposite the interval between the cartilages of the fifth and sixth ribs on the left side, is enclosed in a serous pericardium, and consists as in other

heart 1d(1)

mammals and in birds of four chambers divided into an upper pair of rather thin-walled auricles which receive blood from the veins and a lower pair of thick-walled ventricles into which the blood is forced and which in turn pump it into the arteries, back flow being prevented by valves, or in lower forms is less perfectly differentiated, having usu. two auricles and one ventricle in reptiles and amphibians and but a single auricle and ventricle in most fishes **b :** a structure in an invertebrate animal functionally analogous to the vertebrate heart: as (1) **:** a contractile ventricle with one to four thin-walled auricles that circulates the body fluid of most mollusks (2) **:** a contractile tube in most arthropods that receives blood from an investing pericardial sinus through openings provided with valves and circulates it forward and peripherally in the body (3) **:** any of a series of paired pulsating anterior blood vessels connecting the main dorsal and ventral blood vessels of certain annelids **c :** BREAST, BOSOM (could have hugged him to my ~ —W.M.Thackeray) **d :** something resembling a heart in shape: (1) **:** a conventionalized representation of a heart (as a decorative figure or a trinket) (2) **:** a red conventionalized figure of a heart stamped on a playing card (3) **:** a heart-shaped block through which a lanyard is reeved to extend stays (4) **:** the heart-shaped part of a pound net placed at the end of the leader to direct fish into the pot (5) **:** a foundry molder's heart-shaped trowel (6) **hearts** *pl but sing in constr* **:** a wood sorrel (*Oxalis montana*) **2 a :** a playing card marked with a conventionalized figure of a heart **b hearts** *pl* **:** the suit comprising cards so marked **c :** an odd bridge trick won or contracted for when hearts are trumps **d hearts** *pl but sing in constr* **:** a game resembling whist in which the object is to avoid taking tricks containing hearts and often other specified cards

from Webster's 3rd

THE UNABRIDGED HEART

3 a (1) **:** the whole personality including intellectual as well as emotional functions or traits (come from the ~ that is gay, warm, friendly, and enthusiastic —Constance Foster) (I say what is in my ~) (deep in your own ~, you share my prejudice —Walter de la Mare) (each man knew in his ~ that it was a lie —L.B.Salomon) (2) *obs* **:** INTELLECT, UNDERSTANDING (3) **:** MEMORY, ROTE — used in the phrase *by heart* (got the whole poem by ~) (knew the town's 500 telephone numbers by ~ —Peg Bracken) (4) **:** OPINION, ATTITUDE, POSTURE — used chiefly in the phrase *change of heart* (two aspects to the Soviet change of ~ on the Austrian treaty —T.P.Whitney) **b** (1) **:** the emotional or moral as distinguished from the intellectual nature **:** CONSCIENCE, CHARACTER, SPIRIT (has a good ~ but a weak head) (who can look into the ~ of a man) (his ~ dictated one course, his reason another) (2) **:** generous disposition **:** SENSIBILITY, COMPASSION, FEELINGS (have you no ~) (Oh, have a ~, lend me a dollar) (3) **:** hardness or flintiness of character or temper **:** unfeeling disposition — usu. used with *have* in negative construction (he loved his wife; he had not the ~ to deny her anything —Clara Morris) (hadn't the ~ . . . to refuse to come —Ellen Glasgow) (4) **:** TEMPERAMENT, DISPOSITION, MOOD (went home with a heavy ~) (are not inclined to regard free-trade agitation with a light ~ —*Dun's Rev.*) (5) **:** GOODWILL, WILLINGNESS, SINCERITY, ZEAL — used chiefly in the phrase *with all my heart* (will do it for you with all my ~) **c :** LOVE, AFFECTIONS (he lost his ~ to her at once) (laid his ~ at her feet) (a free public-school system . . . was one thing that lay near his ~ —A.W.Long) (his speeches won him ~*s* from coast to coast —William Clark) **d :** COURAGE, ARDOR, ENTHUSIASM (don't lose ~; all will turn out well) (felt some sinking of the ~) (an unsatisfactory . . . student, for my ~ was not in it —W.S.Maugham) (put ~ into me by what you say —O.W.Holmes †1935) (at the sight of reinforcements, the dispirited soldiers took ~) (lost all ~ for my silly chase —Arthur Grimble) (many a people has kept itself in ~ when its statesmen have despaired —W.B.Adams) **e** (1) **:** TASTE, LIKING (likes music but has no ~ for grand opera) — used chiefly in the phrase *after one's own heart* (a man after his own ~) (2) **:** fixed purpose or desire **:** ardent wish — now used chiefly in the phrase *set one's heart on* (set his ~ on getting a new car) (3) **:** intense concern, solicitude, or preoccupation — used chiefly in the phrase *at heart* (people who are unaware of the issue which he has at ~ —J.H.Robinson) (with victory secured, there was one other thing that he had at ~) **f :** one's innermost being **:** one's innermost or actual character, disposition, or feelings — used chiefly in the phrases *at heart* (at ~ a sensitive high-strung man) and *heart of hearts* (assisting those who in their ~ of hearts are . . . implacably anti-American —Perry Miller) (in his ~ of hearts I do not think he ever really surrenders faith —Edward Wagenknecht) **4 :** PERSON (two young ~*s* had been freed . . . from the burden of guilt and suspicion —Agnes S. Turnbull) — usu. used with a qualifier (poor ~! who would relieve her wants now) (farewell, dear ~) **5 :** the central or decisive part of something **:** CENTER: as **a :** an inner central area or region (a system of waterways extending into the ~ of No. America) **b :** an essential part **:** the part that determines the real nature of something or gives significance to the other parts **:** the determining aspect (the discernment and understanding with which he penetrates to the ~ and essence of the problem —B.N.Cardozo) (those words of Jesus show us the ~ of Easter's meaning —W.F.Hambly) **c :** the center of activity **:** a vital part on which continuing activity or existence depends (Rome was the ~ and pulse of the empire —John Buchan) **d :** HEARTWOOD **e :** CORE 1h **f :** a firm part (as of a head of lettuce); *also* **:** the center of a celery plant **6** *chiefly Brit* **:** condition for bearing crops **:** FERTILITY — used chiefly in the phrase *in good heart* (the land has never been in better ~ —S.P.B.Mais) **syn** see CENTER — **to heart**

adv : under serious consideration : with deep concern : with hurt feelings ⟨took it *to heart*⟩ ⟨Sterne . . . laid the criticism *to heart* —Virginia Woolf⟩ — **to one's heart's content** : to the point of complete satisfaction or satiety : to the limits of one's will or pleasure ⟨eat *to your heart's content*⟩ ⟨printers imported any foreign books they thought would be popular . . . and reprinted them *to their heart's content* —Margaret Nicholson⟩

²**heart** \"\ *vb* -ED/-ING/-S [ME *herten,* fr. OE *hiertan,* fr. *heorte,* n.] *vt* **1** *archaic* : to give heart to : HEARTEN, ENCOURAGE, INSPIRIT **2** : to fix or seat in the heart **3** : to fill in (as a wall) with rubble or similar material ~ *vi* : to form a compact center or heart; *specif* : to develop a head (as of lettuce and cabbage)

³**heart** \"\ *dial var of* HEARTH

heart·ache \ˈ=ˌ=\ *n* : anguish of mind **syn** see SORROW

heart and soul *adv* : without reservations : COMPLETELY, WHOLLY ⟨count on me to help *heart and soul*⟩

heart attack *n* **1** : HEART FAILURE **2** : a seizure of weak or abnormal functioning of the heart

heart balm *n* : compensation for breach of promise to marry or alienation of affections ⟨two days after the marriage . . . was sued by another woman for two hundred thousand dollars' *heart balm* —Carey McWilliams⟩

heart·beat \ˈ=ˌ=\ *n* **1** : one complete pulsation of the heart **2** : the vital center or driving impulse ⟨the dining car is the real ~ and life of a train —Richard Barnitz⟩ ⟨the school is the ~ of our organic society —Agnes Meyer⟩

heart block *n* : incoordination of the heartbeat in which the auricles and ventricles beat independently due to defective transmission through the atrioventricular bundle and marked by decreased cardiac output often with cerebral ischemia

heart bond *n* : a masonry bond in which no header stone stretches across the wall but two headers meet in the middle and their joint is covered by another stone

¹**heartbreak** \ˈ=ˌ=\ *n* **1** : crushing grief ⟨the sorrow and the ~ which . . . abide in the homes of so many of our neighbors —H.S.Truman⟩ **2** : something that causes heartbreak ⟨proved a . . . ~ to the authors of his being —C.G.Glover⟩ ⟨the spectacle of his gentle fortitude was . . . a ~ —John Buchan⟩

²**heartbreak** \"\ *vt* [back-formation fr. *heartbroken*] : to break the heart of

heart·breaker \ˈ=ˌ==\ *n* : something that causes heartbreak ⟨arming merchant ships . . . has been another ~ —Fortune⟩

heart·breaking \ˈ=ˌ==\ *adj* : causing overpowering or intense sorrow, anguish, or distress ⟨made progress only with the most ~ efforts —Farley Mowat⟩ ⟨it is ~ to see new schools going up without proper . . . planning —Cecile Starr⟩ — **heart·break·ing·ly** *adv*

heartbroken \ˈ=ˌ==\ *adj* [¹*heart* + *broken*] : overcome by sorrow — **heart·bro·ken·ly** *adv* — **heart·bro·ken·ness** \ˈhärt-ˌbrōkən(n)ə̇s\ *n* -ES

heartburn \ˈ=ˌ=\ *n* **1** : a burning discomfort behind the lower part of the sternum usu. related to spasm of the lower end of the esophagus or of the cardia of the stomach — called also *cardialgia, pyrosis* **2** : HEARTBURNING

heartburning \ˈ=ˌ==\ *n* : intense or rancorous jealousy or resentment ⟨his promotion to ministerial rank is bound to cause much ~ —J.A.Stevenson⟩ ⟨the seniority rule . . . prevents bitter personal rivalries, factional sniping, and ~ —S.D. Bailey⟩

heart cherry *n* : any of several cultivated sweet cherries with rather soft-fleshed heart-shaped fruits — compare BIGARREAU CHERRY, DUKE 5

heart cockle *n* : ²COCKLE 1a; *esp* : a widely distributed burrowing cockle (*Isocardia cor*) with the umbones well separated giving the shell a heart-shaped appearance

heart disease *n* : an abnormal organic condition of the heart or of the heart and circulation

heart·ed \ˈhärd·ə̇d, ˈhȧ-, ˌtə̇d\ *adj* [ME *herted,* fr. *hert* heart + *-ed* — more at HEART] **1** : having a (specified kind of) heart — often used in combination ⟨gave pleasure to lighter‑*hearted* members of the staff —J.G.Cozzens⟩ **2** : seated or laid up in the heart

heart·ed·ness *n* -ES : the condition of having a heart esp. of a specified kind — often used in combination ⟨hard*heartedness*⟩ ⟨cold*heartedness*⟩

heart block *n* : incoordination of the heartbeat in which the auricles and ventricles beat independently due to defective transmission through the atrioventricular bundle and marked by decreased cardiac output often with cerebral ischemia

heart bond *n* : a masonry bond in which no header stone stretches across the wall but two headers meet in the middle and their joint is covered by another stone

¹**heartbreak** \ˈ=ˌ=\ *n* **1** : crushing grief ⟨the sorrow and the ~ which . . . abide in the homes of so many of our neighbors —H.S.Truman⟩ **2** : something that causes heartbreak ⟨proved a . . . ~ to the authors of his being —C.G.Glover⟩ ⟨the spectacle of his gentle fortitude was . . . a ~ —John Buchan⟩

²**heartbreak** \"\ *vt* [back-formation fr. *heartbroken*] : to break the heart of

heart·breaker \ˈ=ˌ==\ *n* : something that causes heartbreak ⟨arming merchant ships . . . has been another ~ —Fortune⟩

heart·breaking \ˈ=ˌ==\ *adj* : causing overpowering or intense

sorrow, anguish, or distress ⟨made progress only with the most ~ efforts —Farley Mowat⟩ ⟨it is ~ to see new schools going up without proper . . . planning —Cecile Starr⟩ — **heart·break·ing·ly** *adv*

heartbroken \ˈ=ˌ==\ *adj* [¹*heart* + *broken*] : overcome by sorrow — **heart·bro·ken·ly** *adv* — **heart·bro·ken·ness** \ˈhärt-ˌbrōkən(n)ə̇s\ *n* -ES

heartburn \ˈ=ˌ=\ *n* **1** : a burning discomfort behind the lower part of the sternum usu. related to spasm of the lower end of the esophagus or of the cardia of the stomach — called also *cardialgia, pyrosis* **2** : HEARTBURNING

heartburning \ˈ=ˌ==\ *n* : intense or rancorous jealousy or resentment ⟨his promotion to ministerial rank is bound to cause much ~ —J.A.Stevenson⟩ ⟨the seniority rule . . . prevents bitter personal rivalries, factional sniping, and ~ —S.D. Bailey⟩

heart cherry *n* : any of several cultivated sweet cherries with rather soft-fleshed heart-shaped fruits — compare BIGARREAU CHERRY, DUKE 5

heart cockle *n* : ²COCKLE 1a; *esp* : a widely distributed burrowing cockle (*Isocardia cor*) with the umbones well separated giving the shell a heart-shaped appearance

heart disease *n* : an abnormal organic condition of the heart or of the heart and circulation

heart·ed \ˈhärd·ə̇d, ˈhȧ-, ˌtə̇d\ *adj* [ME *herted,* fr. *hert* heart + *-ed* — more at HEART] **1** : having a (specified kind of) heart — often used in combination ⟨gave pleasure to lighter‑*hearted* members of the staff —J.G.Cozzens⟩ **2** : seated or laid up in the heart

heart·ed·ness *n* -ES : the condition of having a heart esp. of a specified kind — often used in combination ⟨hard*heartedness*⟩ ⟨cold*heartedness*⟩

heart·en \ˈhärt²n, ˈhȧt-\ *vb* **heartened**; **heartened**; **hearten·ing** \-t(²)niŋ\ **heartens** [¹*heart-* + *-en*] *vt* **1** : to give heart to : inspire with fresh zeal, hope, or courage : rouse from indifference or discouragement ⟨people . . . whose presence either ~ed the spirit or kindled the mind —Jan Struther⟩ ⟨their supporters are enormously ~ed —Mollie Panter‑Downes⟩ **2** *archaic* : to restore fertility or strength to (as land) ~ *vi* : to take courage : become imbued with fresh spirit and energy ⟨then the engine would ~ up and show off its paces —William Baucke⟩ **syn** see ENCOURAGE

heartening *adj* : tending or serving to hearten, inspire, or give fresh courage ⟨a ~ sign⟩ ⟨a ~ development⟩ — **heart·en·ing·ly** *adv*

heart failure *n* **1** : a condition in which the heart is unable to pump blood at an adequate rate or in adequate volume — see CONGESTIVE HEART FAILURE, CORONARY FAILURE **2** : cessation of the heartbeat : DEATH **3** : a sudden feeling of faintness (as at a surprise or sudden shock)

heartfelt \ˈ=ˌ=\ *adj* : profoundly felt : EARNEST ⟨~ sympathy⟩ ⟨~ thanks⟩ **syn** see SINCERE

heart-free \ˈ=ˌ=\ *adj* : not committed or engaged in one's affections ⟨quite *heart-free* —George Meredith⟩

heart·ful \ˈhärtfəl\ *adj* [ME *hertful,* fr. *hert* heart + *-ful* — more at HEART] : full of heartfelt emotion : HEARTY ⟨~ prayers⟩ — **heart·ful·ly** \-fəlē\ *adv*

heartier *comparative of* HEARTY

heartiest *superlative of* HEARTY

heart·i·ly \ˈhärd·ə̇lē, ˈhȧ-, ˌtə̇-, -li\ *adv* [ME *hertily,* fr. *herty* hearty + *-ly*] **1** : in a hearty manner **2 a** : with all sincerity or goodwill : without reservations : WHOLEHEARTEDLY ⟨~ in sympathy with the essence of the liberal faith —M.R.Cohen⟩ **b** : with zest or gusto : VIGOROUSLY ⟨threw himself ~ into his work⟩ ⟨ate and drank ~⟩ **3** : COMPLETELY, THOROUGHLY, EXCEEDINGLY ⟨~ sick of this idle debate⟩

heart·i·ness \ˌd·ēnə̇s, ˌd·in-\ *n* -ES **1** : cordiality or geniality of manner : CHEERINESS, FRIENDLINESS ⟨detested his backslapping ~⟩ **2** : ZEAL, ENTHUSIASM ⟨the music was sung with uninhibited ~ by the mountain folk —Herman Wouk⟩ ⟨enjoy themselves . . . with a ~ that makes the Londoner feel extremely envious —S.P.B.Mais⟩ **3** : VIGOR, STRENGTH ⟨an air of rugged outdoor ~ —J.J.Godwin⟩

hearting *n* -s [fr. gerund of ²*heart*] **1** : CORE 11 **2** : PUDDLE WALL **3** : BACKING 1a

heart·land \ˈhärt,land, ˈhȧt-, -,laa(ə)nd, -,lənd\ *n* : an area of decisive importance : a pivotal or nuclear area ⟨the entire ~ of the country, the Mississippi Basin —A.W.Baum⟩ ⟨the German industrial ~ in the Ruhr valley —Henry Wallace⟩ ⟨the temperate highlands which are the ~ of the republic — A.P.Whitaker⟩ ⟨the ~ of Eastern duck and goose shooting — Newsweek⟩; *specif* : a central land area (as northern Eurasia from the Elbe to the Amur) conceived by geopoliticians to be capable of self-sufficiency as an economic and military unit, invulnerable to sea power, and therefore having strategic advantages for mastery of the world

heartleaf \ˈ=ˌ=\ *n* : any of several wild gingers that have distinctly cordate leaves and are usu. included in the genus *Asarum* but are sometimes segregated in a separate genus

heart-leaved aster \ˈ=ˌ=-\ *n* : a common blue aster (*Aster cordifolius*) of eastern No. America

heart-leaved willow *also* **heart-leafed willow** \ˈ=ˌ=-\ *n* : a common broad-leaved American willow (*Salix cordata*) with cordate leaves

heart·less \ˈhärtlə̇s, ˈhȧt-\ *adj* [ME *hertles,* fr. *hert* heart +

-*les* -less] **1** : devoid of heart **2** *archaic* : lacking courage or zeal : SPIRITLESS, DESPONDENT   **b** : lacking feeling or affection : UNSYMPATHETIC, CRUEL ⟨it seems so ~ to leave her —G.B. Shaw⟩ ⟨a ~ mother, a false wife —W.M.Thackeray⟩ — **heart·less·ly** *adv* — **heart·less·ness** *n* -ES

heart line *n, usu cap* H : LINE OF HEART

heart liverleaf *or* **heart liverwort** *n* : a hepatica (*Hepatica triloba*)

heart-lung machine *n* : a mechanical pump that shunts the body's blood away from the heart and maintains the circulation during heart surgery

heart murmur *n* : MURMUR 4

heartnut \'ˌˌ·ˌ\ *n* : JAPANESE WALNUT

heart of palm : the edible young terminal bud of various palms (as a cabbage palmetto) usu. served raw and dressed as a salad

heartpea \'ˌˌ·\ *n* [so called fr. the shape of the seed] : BALLOON VINE

heart pine *n* : LONGLEAF PINE

heart rate *n* : a measure of cardiac activity usu. expressed as number of beats per minute

heartrending \'ˌˌˌˌ\ *adj* : causing intense grief, anguish, or pain ⟨gives a ~ description of his own days under a private tutor — G.G.Coveton⟩ ⟨his untimely death was . . . ~ —*Nation*⟩

heart·rend·ing·ly *adv* : in a heartrending manner

heartrot \'ˌˌ·\ *n* : any of several rots involving the central part of a plant or plant organ: as   **a** : disintegration of the heartwood of a tree (as by fungi of the genus *Fomes*)   **b** : a disease of beets and rutabagas caused by a fungus (*Mycosphaerella tabifica*) that brings about decay of the heart and blighting of the leaves   **c** : a rot of sugar beets caused by boron deficiency

hearts *pl of* HEART, *pres 3d sing of* HEART

heart sac *n* : PERICARDIUM

hearts-and-flowers *n pl but sing or pl in constr* : show of sentiment or sentimentality ⟨cloying expressions of endearment ⟨cut out the *hearts-and-flowers* —Maritta Wolff⟩ ⟨I can't stand *hearts-and-flowers* stuff —Mary Miller⟩

heart-scalded \'hˌärtˌskȯdˌəd\ *adj, dial Brit* : tormented by sorrow or remorse : TROUBLED

heart-searching \'ˌˌˌˌ\ *n* : introspective analysis or self-examination ⟨the decision was reached only after prolonged *heart-searching* —*Times Lit. Supp.*⟩ ⟨of course these choices will not have been made without *heart-searchings* and reservations —A.J.Toynbee⟩

hearts·ease \'hˌürtˌsēz, 'hát-\ *n* [ME *herts ese*, fr. *herts* (gen. of *hert* heart) + *ese* ease] **1** : peace of mind : TRANQUILLITY ⟨religion failed to bring him ~ —R.H.Bainton⟩ **2 a** : any of various violas: as (1) : WILD PANSY (2) : a common Old World viola (*Viola arvensis*) with creamy often violet-tinged flowers (3) : a violet (*V. ocellata*) of the Pacific coast of No. America with white petals tinged or marked with yellow and deep violet   **b** : any of several smartweeds   **3** : a strong violet that is redder and paler than pansy or clematis and redder and lighter than royal purple (sense 2)

heartseed \'ˌˌ·\ *n* [so called fr. the heart-shaped white spot on the black seed] : a plant of the genus *Cardiospermum*; *esp* : BALLOON VINE

heart shake *n* : a defect in timber consisting of shrinkage and separation of tissues across the annual rings usu. along the rays — compare RING SHAKE

heart shell *n* **1** : any of numerous bivalve mollusks esp. of the families Cardiidae and Carditidae with shells that are heart-shaped in outline when viewed from the end   **2** : the shell of a heart-shell mollusk

heartsick \'ˌˌ·\ *adj* : very despondent : DEPRESSED ⟨was too ~ to rise and fight —W.A.White⟩ : reflecting or marked by a feeling of sickness ⟨longed with a ~ yearning for the first few days to be over —W.M.Thackeray⟩

heartsickening *adj* : causing depression or despondency

heartsickness \'ˌˌˌˌ\ *n* : the quality or state of being heartsick ⟨died of . . . ~ after moving here and waiting for years for the man who never came —*Nat'l Geographic*⟩ ⟨the wild ~ of the desert —Lawrence Durrell⟩

heart snakeroot *n* [so called fr. the shape of the leaf] : WILD GINGER 2a

heart·some \'hˌertsəm\ *adj* ['heart + -*some*] *chiefly Scot* : animating and enlivening : giving cheer ⟨a ~ thing, the smell of frying ham on a frosty morning —G.D.Brown⟩ — **heart·some·ly** *adv*

heartsore \'ˌˌ·\ *adj* : HEARTSICK ⟨a ~ lover⟩

heartstring \'ˌˌˌ\ *n* [ME *hertstring*, fr. *hert* heart + *string*] **1** *obs* : a nerve or tendon supposed to support or sustain the heart   **2** : the deepest emotions or affections — usu. used in pl. ⟨tore at the ~s of memory —William Beebe⟩ ⟨could touch the ~s of the audience —E.H.Collis⟩

heart-struck \'ˌˌˌ\ *adj* **1** : struck to the heart   **2** *archaic* : driven to the heart : infixed in the mind

heartthrob \'ˌˌˌ\ *n* **1** : the throb of a heart   **2 a** : sentimental emotion : PASSION ⟨diary of ~s and rebuffs —*New Republic*⟩   **b** : SWEETHEART ⟨a girl on the . . . verge of giving her ~ the raspberry —P.G.Wodehouse⟩

heart tie *n* : a railroad crosstie with sapwood one fourth or less the width of the tie at the top measured at a point 20 inches to 40 inches from the middle of the tie

heart-to-heart \'ˌˌˌˌ\ *adj* : SINCERE, FRANK ⟨a *heart-to-heart* talk⟩

heart trefoil *n* [so called fr. the shape of the leaves] : SPOTTED MEDIC

heart urchin *n* : a heart-shaped sea urchin

heart wall *n* : CORE 11

heartwarming \'ˌˌˌˌ\ *adj* : inspiring a glow of sympathetic feeling : pleasantly moving or stirring : CHEERING ⟨her story of their experiences is entertaining and ~ —*Huntting's Monthly List*⟩ ⟨most ~ literary event of the year —*New Internat'l Yr. Bk.*⟩

heartwater \'ˌˌˌˌ\ *n* [so called fr. the accumulation of fluid in the pericardium] : a serious febrile disease of sheep, goats, and cattle in southern Africa caused by a rickettsial microorganism (*Cowdria ruminantium*) transmitted by a tick (*Amblyomma hebraeum*)

heartweed \'ˌˌˌ\ *n* : LADY'S THUMB

heart-whole \'ˌˌˌ\ *adj* **1** : not broken or depressed in spirit : UNDISMAYED ⟨so many clowns have been small . . . pathetic; here is one large and *heart-whole* —G.W.Stonier⟩ **2** : having the affections free : not in love   **3** : free from deceit or hypocrisy : SINCERE, GENUINE ⟨a *heart-whole* friendship —George Meredith⟩

heartwise \'hˌürt,wīz\ *adv* ['heart + -*wise*] : in the shape or manner of a heart ⟨her face . . . tapered ~ —T.B.Costain⟩

heartwood \'ˌˌˌ\ *n* : the older harder nonliving central portion of wood usu. being darker in color, denser, less permeable, and more durable than the surrounding sapwood but in some woods (as white spruce) lacking distinctive color and then being difficult to distinguish — called also *duramen*

heartworm \'ˌˌˌ\ *n* **1** : a filarial worm (*Dirofilaria immitis*) that is esp. common in warm regions, lives as an adult in the right heart of dogs and some other carnivores, and discharges active larvae into the circulating blood whence they may be picked up by mosquitoes and transmitted to other hosts   **2** : infestation with or disease caused by the heartworm resulting typically in gasping, coughing, and nervous disorder and when severe commonly leading to death

hearty \'hˌürt|dˌē, 'hˌä|, |tˌē, -i\ *adj* -ER/-EST [ME *herty*, fr. *hert* heart + -*y*] **1 a** : giving unqualified support : unreservedly loyal : THOROUGHGOING, ENTHUSIASTIC ⟨a ~ Federalist —F.J. Klingberg⟩ ⟨a ~ assumer of its full share of . . . responsibilities —F.S.C.Northrop⟩ ⟨my ~ concurrence in everything you've done —T.B.Costain⟩   **b** (1) : exuberantly or unreservedly cordial or genial : not reserved or ceremonious in manner : JOVIAL ⟨had a bluff and ~ bearing, but he was a rogue —Ross Annett⟩ ⟨being a shade too ~ about it —Angus Mowat⟩ ⟨a wonderful ~ manner with a boy —G.D.Brown⟩ (2) : giving exuberant or unrestrained expression to one's feelings ⟨a ~ burst of laughter greeted his arrival⟩ ⟨a string of ~ curses⟩ (3) : APPROVING ⟨no one but a Chancery lawyer had a ~ word for the Chancery —F.W.Maitland⟩ ⟨some colleagues are distinctly less ~ about the General —Hal Lehrman⟩ **2 a** : exhibiting vigorous good health ⟨the mate was as ~ as a young lion —Herman Melville⟩ ⟨is my friend ~, now I am thin and pine —A.E.Housman⟩   **b** (1) : having a good appetite : consuming abundantly or with gusto ⟨a ~ eater⟩ ⟨a ~ drinker⟩ (2) : ABUNDANT, AMPLE ⟨ate a ~ meal⟩ ⟨took a ~ swig⟩   **c** : NOURISHING, INVIGORATING ⟨almost a meal in itself, with 15 tender vegetables in ~ beef stock —*Better Homes & Gardens*⟩ ⟨has a ~ flavor that is much livelier than our refined . . . variety —Silas Spitzer⟩ : FULL-BODIED ⟨a ~ Rhone with a full bouquet —*New Yorker*⟩   **3** : vigorous or violent in manner or degree : VEHEMENT ⟨the breeze . . . was *heartier* . . . than before —Llewellyn Howland⟩ ⟨hooked a root and gave a ~ pull —C.S.Forester⟩ ⟨then came the rain in a ~ flood —John Muir †1914⟩ ⟨the wind had combed up some quite ~ waves —R.A.W.Hughes⟩ ⟨without any provocation at all give him a ~ kick —H.A.Chippendale⟩ **4** *chiefly Brit* : capable of bearing crops : FERTILE ⟨thistles so growing . . . signifieth the land to be ~ —Thomas Tusser⟩ *syn* see SINCERE

²hearty \'\ *n* -ES : a bold brave fellow : COMRADE — used esp. in addressing sailors ⟨heave-ho, my *hearties*⟩   **b** : SAILOR ⟨the albatross mocked by the *hearties* —Stephen Spender⟩ **2** *chiefly Brit* : an individual of exuberant outgoing disposition or of athletic nonaesthetic tastes ⟨a Matisse reproduction could cause one's rooms to be wrecked . . . by rugger *hearties* —Jocelyn Brooke⟩

heart yarn *n* : yarn in the center of a rope

heart 1d(1)

A Heart at Rest

When the voices of children are
heard on the green
And laughing is heard on the hill,
My heart is at rest within my breast
And everything else is still.
—William Blake

HEART ROOTS

English-language words that are related historically to the word heart come to us from three main linguistic branches. These all have a common origin in Indo-European, the hypothetical mother tongue of many of the world's languages. Thus the postulated Indo-European form *kerd,* meaning heart, branched out into several directions, giving rise to the proto-heart word in the Germanic, the Hellenic, and the Italic tongues.

From the Germanic stem *herton* we derive our modern term and all its obvious relatives. From the Hellenic *kardia* (heart, stomach, spirit, ego) we get scientific terms such as cardiac, pericardium, and a host of other anatomical variations. From the Italic branch, via the Latin *cor* (heart), we derive such words as cordial, courage, discord, and record, all having some concept of heart at their root. Our verb "record," for example, comes from the Latin *re-cordari,* meaning "to remember"; the derivation implies that the act of remembering was originally considered a function of the heart—we do learn things "by heart"—and this is consistent with the frequent use in many older languages of a single word for both the mental and emotional functions.

Other offshoots of the Indo-European *kerd* made comparatively few contributions to the English vocabulary. One isolated example is the word "machree," which comes via the Celtic branch from the Old Irish *cride* (heart). This form evolved into the later Irish *mo chroidhe* (my heart) and finally gave rise to machree, a term of endearment now used in the sense of "my dear."

Her heart, like the lake,
  was as pure and as calm,
Till love o'er it came,
  like a breeze o'er the sea,
And made the heart heave
  of sweet Mary machree.
  —Samuel Lover

20

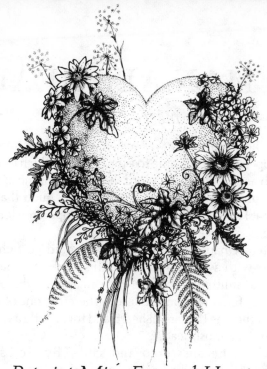

Betwixt Mine Eye and Heart

William Shakespeare

Betwixt mine eye and heart a league is took,
And each doth good turns now unto the other:
When that mine eye is famish'd for a look,
Or heart in love with sighs himself doth smother,
With my love's picture then my eye doth feast,
And to the painted banquet bids my heart;
Another time mine eye is my heart's guest,
And in his thoughts of love doth share a part.
So either by thy picture or my love,
Thyself away are present still with me,
For thou not farther than my thoughts canst move,
And I am still with them, and they with thee;
    Or if they sleep, thy picture in my sight
    Awakes my heart to heart's and eye's delight.

A MAN ALL HEART

a merry old tale

A northern man there was which went to seek him a service. So it happened that he came to a lord's place, which lord then had war with another lord. This lord then asked this northern man if that he durst fight. "Yea, by God's bones," quod that northern man, "that I dare, for I is all heart." Whereupon the lord retained him into his service.

So after, it happened that his lord should go fight with his enemies, with whom also went this northern man—which shortly was smitten in the heel with an arrow, wherefore he incontinently fell down almost dead. Wherefore one of his fellows said: "Art thou he that art all heart, and for so little a stroke in the heel now art almost dead?"

To whom he answered and said: "By God's soul I is heart—head, legs, body, heels, and all—therefore ought not one to fear when he is stricken in the heart?"

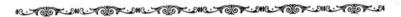

The Allegory of the Body and the Heart

An Arthurian Vignette, by Chretien de Troyes

"My heart is wax molded as she pleases, but enduring as marble to retain."—Cervantes

"There is no feeling in a human heart which exists in that heart alone—which is not, in some form or degree, in every heart."
—George MacDonald

"The great man is he who does not lose his child's-heart."—Mencius

"My lord Yvain is so distressed to leave his lady that his heart remains behind. The King may take his body off, but he cannot lead his heart away. She who stays behind clings so tightly to his heart that the King has not the power to take it away with him. When the body is left without the heart it cannot possibly live on. For such a marvel was never seen as the body alive without the heart. Yet this marvel now came about: for he kept his body without the heart, which was wont to be enclosed in it, but which would not follow the body now. The heart has a good abiding-place, while the body, hoping for a safe return to its heart, in strange fashion takes a new heart of hope, which is so often deceitful and treacherous."

LITERARY QUIZ

Match the titles of the following literary works with their authors.

1. *The Heart Keeper*   a. Nathaniel West

2. *The Heart of Man*   b. Conrad Aiken

3. *The Heart of Midlothain*   c. Carson McCullers

4. *In the Heart of the*
   Heart of the Country   d. Francoise Sagan

5. *Hearts of the West*   e. Mikhail Bulgakov

6. *The Heart of the Matter*   f. Dee Brown

7. *Heartbreak House*   g. Joseph Conrad

8. *Heart of Darkness*   h. Erich Fromm

9. *The Heart is*
   a Lonely Hunter   i. Belasco & Hearne

10. *The Heart of a Dog*   j. Sir Walter Scott

11. *A Heart for the*
    Gods of Mexico   k. Graham Greene

12. *Bury My Heart*
    at Wounded Knee   l. George Bernard Shaw

13. *Hearts of Oak*   m. William Gass

14. *Miss Lonelyhearts*   n. O. Henry

"Open my heart, and you will see
Graved inside of it, 'Italy.'"
—Robert Browning

Like most parents, in my heart of hearts I have a
favorite child. That child is David Copperfield.
—Charles Dickens

"It is the writer's privilege to help man endure by
lifting his heart."—William Faulkner

ANSWERS: (1), d; (2), h; (3), j; (4), m; (5), n; (6), k; (7), l; (8), g; (9), c; (10), e; (11), b; (12), f; (13), i; (14), a.

The title poem of W.D. Snodgrass's Pulitzer Prize winning book *Heart's Needle* (1959) was adapted from the old Irish saying that *An only daughter is the needle of the heart.*

ST. VALENTINE'S DAY

St. Valentine's Day can be traced back to several different kinds of celebrations that were all held on or about the fourteenth of February. Gradually, they were absorbed into a unique holiday that borrowed from each festival.

The oldest of these is the Roman feast of the Lupercalia, which was held as far back as the third century B.C. in honor of the god Lupercus, protector of shepherds and their flocks. When Christianity became the prevailing religion, many popular pagan holidays were transformed into religious holidays, and pagan gods were replaced by Christian saints. Thus the Lupercalia became St. Valentine's Day, in remembrance of several Christians of that name who had been martyred by the Romans.

So the date of the holiday comes from the Romans, and the name from the early Christians, but what about its close identification with lovers? This seems to have begun with legends that credited the early martyrs with earthly as well as spiritual love. Over the years, they became not only examples of religious fortitude but patrons of lovers as well.

During the Middle Ages, many folk customs began to be associated with St. Valentine's Day. There was, for instance, the very old belief that the birds chose their mates on February fourteenth. From this came the practice in which all the unmarried men and women of a community drew the names of their "valentines" out of a box. This did not mean that a man and a woman would become sweethearts, but it did oblige the man to wear his valentine's name on his sleeve and serve as her protector during the next year.

From the selection of valentines, it was only a short step to the exchange of presents. And it stands to reason that the heart—symbol for thousands of years of love, fidelity, and honesty—should be used in these gifts as the symbol most appropriate to the day.

The heart and the eyes, explains the troubadour poet Aimeric de Peguilhan, are the organs of love: *"True Love, I assure you, has not, and cannot have of himself, force or power, or any authority either small or great, unless the eyes and the heart give it to him. . . . For the eyes are the dragoman of the heart, and the eyes seek out what it pleases the heart to retain; and when they are well accorded all three, and firmly of one mind, then True Love is born from that which the eyes make pleasing to the heart. . . . And so, let all true lovers know that Love is a true affection which is born of the heart and of the eyes, without doubt, that the eyes make it flower and the heart causes it to bear fruit—Love, the fruit of the true seed."*

"The heart is a brittle thing, and one false vow can break it."—E.G. Bulwer-Lytton

When a young man complains that a young lady has no heart, it is a pretty certain sign that she has his.—George D. Prentice

24

"The heart in itself is not the beginning of life; but it is a vessel formed of thick muscle, vivified and nourished by the artery and vein as are the other muscles."

"Of the heart: This moves of itself and does not stop unless for ever."

—Leonardo da Vinci

A RENAISSANCE HEART

Leonardo Da Vinci, artist, architect, inventor, perhaps the greatest of all the great men of the Renaissance, was also a tireless student of the human body. A superb, self-trained anatomist, he made many original contributions to the field. While every part of the body held his fascination and received his close attention, he came back to the study of the heart again and again.

He compared the heart and its importance to the earth.

"The lake of blood that lies about the heart is the ocean. Its breathing is by the increase and decrease of the blood in its pulses, and even so in the earth is the ebb and flow of the sea. And the vital heat of the world is fire which is spread throughout the world . . . ."

On this matter of heat, it was Leonardo's belief that the temperature of the blood was kept warm by

"the movement of the heart, and this manifests itself because in proportion as the heart moves more swiftly the heat increases more, as is shown by the pulse of those suffering from fever which is moved by the beating of the heart."

He was wrong in this, but he would have needed much more sophisticated medical equipment than any in existence at that time to discover the more subtle causes of body temperature.

Leonardo also noted that the heart carried on its action independent of any action of man. And he noted that:

"The heart . . . moves three thousand five hundred and forty times in each hour in the process of opening and shutting. And it is this frequency of movement which warms the thick muscles of the heart, and this heat warms the blood that continually beats within it. It heats it more in the left ventricle, where the walls are very thick, than in the right ventricle, with the thin wall. And this heat makes the blood grow thinner and turns it to vapor and changes it into air, and would change it to elemental fire, if it were not that the lung renders help at this crisis with the coolness of its air."

The fourteenth-century alchemist and physician Paracelsus believed that the heart heated the rest of the body.

25

WHAT'S A HEART LIKE?

Perhaps it would be easier to say what the heart is *not* like, for the diversity of things to which the heart has been compared does more than tickle the imagination: it courts it. And once the imagination is seduced, anything may happen. For example:

"A woman's heart is as intricate as a ravelled skein of silk."
—*Pere Dumas*

"The human heart is like Indian rubber: a little swells it, but a great deal will not burst it."—*Anne Bronte*

"My heart is like fire in a close vessel: I am ready to burst for want of vent."—*John Wesley*

"A maiden's heart is as champagne, ever struggling upward."
—*C.S. Calverley*

"The heart of a man has been compared to flowers; but unlike them, it does not wait for the blowing of the wind to be scattered abroad."—*Yohida Kenko*

"The hearts of pretty women, like New Year's bonbons, are wrapped in enigmas."—*J. Petit-Senn*

"The heart of a man is like a delicate weed,
That requires to be trampled on boldly indeed."—*Anon.*

"The heart is like an instrument whose strings steal nobler music from life's many frets."—*Gerald Massey*

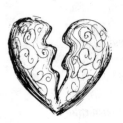

My heart is like a singing bird
 Whose nest is in a watered shoot;
My heart is like an apple-tree
 Whose boughs are bent with thickset fruit;
My heart is like a rainbow shell
 That paddles in a halcyon sea;
My heart is gladder than all these
 Because my love is come to me.
—Christina Rossetti

"The heart is a viper, hissing, and spitting poison at God."—Jonathon Edwards

❦❦❦❦❦❦❦❦

TRAEH?

In their spare time, secretaries at the G. & C. Merriam Company, publishers of Merriam-Webster Reference Books, index *backwards* entries from their Third New International Unabridged Dictionary. To whom might this backward file, as they call it, be of use? Well, some people just can't resist reading a new detective novel from the end forward; and others—an insatiable cardiophile, for example—may simply enjoy perusing an authoritative list of English terms and phrases ending with the word heart. Notice the (reverse) alphabetical sequence in the list which G. & C. Merriam kindly furnished us:

heart	demerara greenheart
septemic heart	broken heart
deadheart	lion heart
red heart	brown heart
cloistered heart	tobacco heart
firm red heart	pseudo-heart
boxed heart	heart-to-heart
round-heart	tiger heart
irritable heart	athlete's heart
purpleheart	bullock's heart
white heart	lion's heart
change of heart	mother's heart
line of heart	soldier's heart
bleeding heart	smoker's heart
floating heart	greatheart
lymph heart	sweetheart
blackheart	left heart
bullock heart	right heart
mechanical heart	faintheart
artificial heart	hollow heart
branchial heart	oxheart
greenheart	pulmonary heart

"The heart of man is made to reconcile contradiction."—David Hume

"So the heart be right, it is no matter which way the head lieth."—Sir Walter Raleigh

27

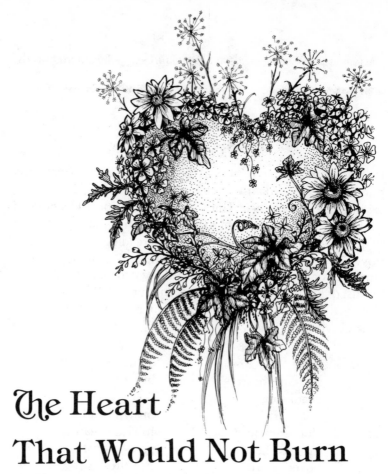

The Heart
That Would Not Burn

Percy Bysshe Shelley, one of England's greatest Romantic poets, drowned when his sailboat sank off the Italian coast in 1822. He was twenty-nine years old.

Shelley's body was recovered and his closest friends, Lord Byron, Leigh Hunt, and Edward Trelawny, arranged to have it cremated. Trelawny's record of the ceremony notes that the fire was fierce, and consumed all of the body but the heart, which he snatched from the flames, severely burning his hand in the process. Leigh Hunt prevailed upon Trelawny to give up the heart, but he in turn was persuaded to turn it over to Shelley's wife, Mary (the author of Frankenstein). Mary never remarried, and through a long life the heart was always with her. Wrapped in silk, it was kept in a special pouch attached to a copy of one of Shelley's volumes of poetry. After her death, it was buried with the body of one of Percy and Mary's sons.

A common superstition among the Romans was the belief that the heart of a person who had been poisoned would not burn. This notion seems to have originated in India and been passed on to the Romans by the Syrians. Germanicus, governor of Syria during the reign of the Emperor Tiberius, died of a prolonged and undiagnosed illness in the year 19 A.D. When his rival and enemy, Piso, was brought to trial, one piece of evidence offered against him was the fact that after Germanicus had been cremated his heart was found whole and unsinged in the ashes.

28

GAME of HEARTS

The game of Hearts was developed in the nineteen twenties. Since then, some twenty different variations on the basic game—such as Joker Hearts, Match Style Hearts, Greek Hearts, and Progressive Hearts—have been developed. The basic rules for the most popular version of Hearts—known as Black Queen, Slippery Anne, or Discard Hearts—are fairly simple, and the most important one to remember is that in Hearts the person with the *lowest* score wins the game.

A standard pack of cards (minus the jokers) is used, and from three to six people may play. The cards are shuffled and then dealt so that each player has the same number. Any that are left over are placed face down in the center of the table and must be collected by the first person to take a heart. Before play begins, each player selects three cards from his hand and passes them, face down, to the player on his left. A player must pass before he can look at the cards he has received from his neighbor.

The player who has been dealt the two of clubs makes the opening lead, and the other players must play cards in the same suit. If they are unable to follow suit, they may discard from any of the others. The ace is high in all suits, with the rest of the cards descending in value in the usual order. The person who has played the highest card in the suit that was led must take the hand.

The objective is to avoid having to take any hearts, since each heart counts for one point. Players also try to avoid the queen of spades, which is worth thirteen points. On the other hand, a daring player with the right hand can attempt to take all the hearts *and* the queen of spades. If he succeeds, all the players receive twenty-six points and he receives none.

There is no standard number of points that constitute a game. Any number of deals may be played before the players agree to stop and add up the score. At this point, the players' individual totals are combined into a grand total. This is then divided by the number of players to determine an average score. Each player who has scored above the average pays into the pot the difference between this average and his own score. Each player having a total score below the average collects the difference between that score and his own from the pot.

Moving Your Heart-ache

It is a common but nonetheless sophisticated observation that if you move an H to the other end of eartH you will discover Heart. And conversely, you may discover the earth in the heart. Shuffle the letters of HEART and see how many other words you can find within it.

ANSWERS: hare, hart, hat, hate, hear, heat, her, rat, rate, rather, tar, tare, tea, tear, the; are, ate; ear, earth, eat.

29

THE HEART-LUNG MACHINE

Open heart surgery, while it is never routine, is regularly and safely carried out many thousands of times each year. But until quite recently, it wasn't possible. Even though surgeons suspected that they could correct many otherwise fatal problems if they had access to the heart, there was no way they could operate on the heart and still maintain its vital functions. Blood must circulate constantly through the body and must be cleansed regularly of its wastes. If the supply of oxygenated blood to the brain is interrupted for as little as four minutes, permanent damage will result.

Designs for a machine that could assume all the heart's functions for short periods of time had been put forward as early as 1885, but the technology to carry them out simply didn't exist. It was not until 1954, following some nineteen years of research and development spearheaded by Dr. John Gibbon, that the first successful heart-lung machine was produced. While the machine is functioning, the surgeon can work uninterrupted on the exposed heart, taking his time to carry out delicate repair work.

The heart-lung machine makes possible a complete cardiopulmonary bypass—all the essential functions of the heart are assumed by the machine. Blood returning to the heart is diverted by means of plastic tubes in the two major veins (the venae cavae) that are responsible for returning blood to the heart. Blood reaching these veins is immediately shunted into the artificial "lung," where carbon dioxide is removed and oxygen is added to the blood. Then the blood is returned to the body via one of the arteries. A pump in the machine supplies just the right amount of pressure to keep the blood circulating through the body at the correct rate. If this rate should be too slow or too fast, the patient could suffer injury and even death. In preventing these occurrences and fulfilling its main function, the heart-lung machine amply demonstrates why almost twenty years of research were needed to produce such a technically sophisticated piece of life-sustaining equipment.

The New York Times has reported that The National Heart, Lung and Blood Institute is conducting a study among thirty institutions to determine whether aspirin can prevent heart attacks by preventing the formation of clots. The Aspirin Myocardial Infarction Study, as it is called, is being sponsored by the Institute to the beat of 17 million dollars.

Reflections on
HEART TRANSPLANTS

"The reality of organ transplants," writes Dr. Shelby D. Gerking, "forces our society to focus on issues that before had been only aimless speculations. Unlike other organs, such as the kidney, the heart is an unpaired structure with little likelihood that the transplant will be made between two individuals in the same family where the immune response is less violent. This situation drastically reduces the number of options open to the surgeon and places him in the unenviable position of choosing the recipient and the donor. The heart of the recipient, while still partially functional, must be judged to be damaged beyond repair; the heart of the donor must be excised immediately after a fatal accident to safeguard the tissue from injury during the interim between removal and transplant. The quick removal of the donor heart has, according to some, demanded a substitute for cardiac arrest as a criterion of death. Our minds are so thoroughly conditioned to equate life with the beating heart that the possibility of using such a heart for transplantation calls into question the very foundations of our legal, moral, and ethical codes. For the time being, we can avoid this confrontation, but the search continues for some method of immobilizing the antibody-producing systems and even constructing a mechanical heart that can be implanted in place of the real thing. As long as man fears death, he will search for ways of prolonging life beyond his appointed years."

The first "successful" heart transplant was done in 1905. Both the donor and the recipient were dogs. After the completed operation, the transplanted heart beat for one hour.

The first heart transplant was performed on Louis Washkansky, 55, at the Groote Schuur Hospital in Capetown, South Africa on December 3, 1967. In a 5 hour operation, Dr. Christiaan Barnard and a team of 30 replaced Washkansky's heart with that of Miss Denise Ann Darvall, 25. Washkansky died 18 days later.

THE PUREST THEATRE

Of all the body's organs, writes surgeon Richard Selzer, "the heart is purest theatre, one is quick to concede, throbbing in its cage palpably as any nightingale. It quickens in response to the emotions. Let danger threaten, and the thrilling heart skips a beat or two and tightrope-walks arrhythmically before lurching back into the forceful thump of fight or flight. And all the while we feel it, hear it even—we, its stage and its audience."

At one time the most popular play on the Peking stage, Red Heart dramatized the story of a group of doctors conducting research in heart disease who overcame harassment by a so-called radical gang of four.

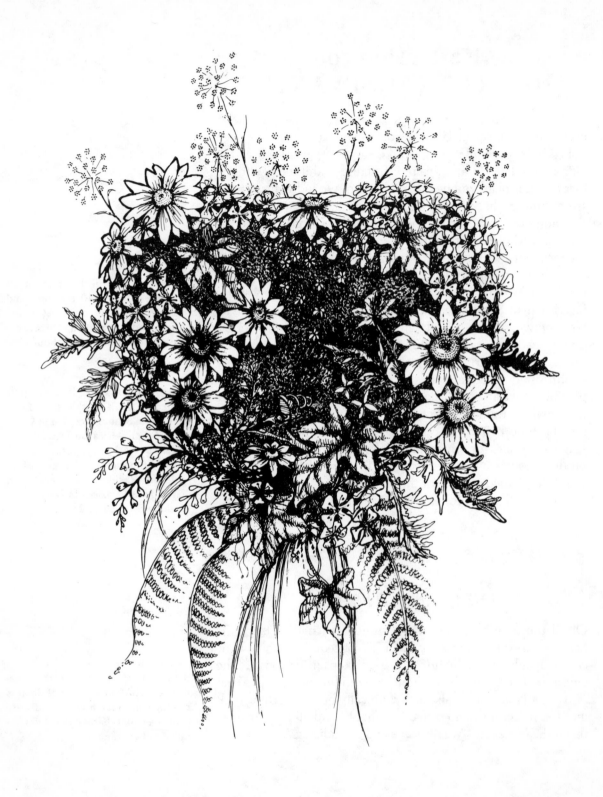

THE
LOST
HEART

a curious historical anecdote

We all of us lose our heart to something or someone at least once in our lives (or, at least, we say we do). Of course, we are speaking metaphorically. There is, however, one exception to this general meaning: the heart of the Marquis of Montrose, preserved after he died, which has been appearing and disappearing, passing from hand to hand, for over three hundred years.

The Marquis had the misfortune of having been on the losing side during the English Civil War. In 1650, he was first hung, and then his body dismembered, the usual fate of those foolish or brave enough to oppose the prevailing power. The Napier family, having among their number several Lords, were Montroses' most faithful friends. Montrose had often promised Lady Napier that when he died she should have his heart. After the burial of the Marquis' body, a friend of the Napier's did, under cover of darkness, exhume the corpse and remove the heart. The organ was embalmed by a "skillful apothecary," wrapped in a coarse cloth, and placed in a small steel case fashioned from the blade of the Marquis' sword. This was in turn placed in a box made of gold and decorated with delicate filigree work, and then, box within box, was deposited in a hefty urn made of silver. Lady Napier kept the urn for some time (indeed, it sat on a table by her bedside). She later sent it to the Marquis' son, then in exile on the continent. Although the young Marquis later returned to the British

The Lost Heart

Isles, he apparently left the urn in the keeping of his good friend, the young Lord Napier, who had elected to stay in Europe. Soon after the friends parted, Lord Napier was robbed, and the golden box stolen.

It was assumed that the box would never be seen again, but in one of the many remarkable coincidences that mark the Montrose story, the box was discovered among the possessions of a collector in Holland—and discovered by a close friend of the Napier family familiar with the story of the heart. He bought it and returned it to the Napiers. Almost a century later, the box and its contents passed into the possession of a Napier daughter, Hester. When she, her husband, and son, took ship for India, as her husband had secured a job in the British administration there, the golden casket went with them. En route, their ship was attacked by a French frigate (at that time, England and France being at war). Hester, her son and husband stayed on deck throughout the action. A shell from the frigate struck a gun, killed several men, and sprayed splinters across the deck. One of the splinters struck the bag in which Hester had collected all her valuables, and which she held at her side. The golden box was destroyed, but the steel container holding the heart was unscratched. In India, Hester's husband hired local goldsmiths to produce a replica of the box, on which the story of Montrose's life and death were engraved in several Indian dialects.

Unfortunately, the box and its contents soon acquired a powerful reputation among the Indian population, as a talisman so effective that whoever possessed it could never be hurt in battle. Inevitably, the casket was stolen, and although it was rumored to have passed into the collection of a local Indian maharajah, nothing could be done to prove this, or to regain it. Almost twenty years later, Hester's son Alexander had occasion to visit the prince reputed to own the box. During a hunt in which both men engaged, Alexander's actions had the effect of allowing the prince to kill a prize boar. In gratitude, the prince asked Alexander what he could do to properly demonstrate his appreciation and regard: Alexander delicately introduced the story of the box and its contents. The prince admitted having the casket, having bought it at a great cost. However, he unhesitantly gave it up, and the heart was once again in the possession of the Napier family.

In 1792 Alexander and his parents set out to return to England.

They traveled across France, and were just about to take ship from Boulogne for home when the Revolutionary government then in power passed a law requiring all gold and silver to be turned over to the state. It seemed impossible to smuggle the golden box past the port authorities, so Hester found an Englishwoman by the name of Knowles living quietly in Boulogne. The box and its contents were given into her possession, until such time as they could be reclaimed. While Hester and her family arrived safely home, any hopes of soon recovering the casket were dashed when war broke out between England and France. It was not until 1815, when a lasting peace was finally secured, that Alexander was able to make the short trip back to Boulogne, to reclaim the Napier treasure. But Mrs. Knowles had died and there was no record of the disposal of her possessions.

The box and its contents have not turned up since. Perhaps, this time, they are really gone, and the heart of Lord Montrose has been cast away on some alien ground. However, considering its unique record of reappearances, it is probably still premature to mark the story "closed." So, if, in a dusty, fly-specked window of some old curiosity shop, on some forgotten street, you catch sight of a dingy casket with strange writing upon it, go in and take it up. And if, inside, you find a steel container the shape and size of an egg, look further. If, in the steel egg, you find a packet wrapped in a rough cloth, with a substance like dried glue spread over it, pay whatever is asked for the casket, for it is likely that you are holding in your hands that elusive prize, the wandering heart of the Marquis of Montrose.

What other dungeon is so dark as one's own heart!
—Nathaniel Hawthorne

Ah, nothing is too late,
Till the tired heart shall cease to palpitate. —H.W. Longfellow

Never morning wore to evening, but some heart did break. —Tennyson

And there is even a happiness
That makes the heart afraid. —Thomas Hood

Hearty Song Titles

A Headache and a Heart
Always in My Heart
Cross Your Heart
Dear Heart
Deep in the Heart of Texas
Don't Go Breaking My Heart
Down in My Heart
Drums in My Heart
Follow Your Heart
Foolish Heart
Give Me a Heart To Sing To
Heart and Soul
Heart—It's a Lovebeat
Heartbreak Hotel
Her Heart Was in Her Work
How Can You Mend a Broken Heart?
I Left My Heart in San Francisco
I Let a Song Go out of My Heart
If You Haven't Got a Sweetheart
I'll Follow My Secret Heart
I've a Strange New Rhythm in My Heart
Let Me Call You Sweetheart
Little More Heart
Love from a Heart of Gold
May Your Heart Stay Young
My Heart Cries for You
My Heart is Full of You
My Heart is Like a Violin
My Heart Leaps Up
My Heart Won't Say Goodbye
My Heart's a Darlin'
My Heart's in the Middle of July
Put a Little Love in Your Heart
Restless Heart
Search Your Heart
Sergeant Pepper's Lonely Heart's Club Band
Sheer Heart Attack
That's When Your Heartache Begins
Way to a Man's Heart
We Will Always Be Sweethearts
When Hearts Are Young
Yes My Heart
You Belong to My Heart
You Set My Heart to Music
Your Cheatin' Heart
You're Breaking My Heart

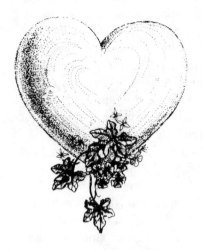
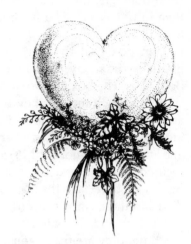

With a Heart in My Song

Match the following heart songs with the recording artists who made them popular.

SONG	ARTIST
1. Cold, Cold Heart	a. Rolling Stones
2. Crazy Heart	b. Mary Martin
3. Heart of My Heart	c. Barbra Streisand
4. Heart of Stone	d. Hank Williams
5. Heart on the Line	e. Peter Frampton
6. My Heart Belongs to Daddy	f. Hill & Range
7. My Heart Belongs to Me	g. Frank Sinatra
8. Peg O' My Heart	h. Hank Williams
9. This Heart of Mine	i. Four Aces
10. Young at Heart	j. Leo Fesit

ANSWERS: (1) d; (2) h; (3) i; (4) a; (5) e; (6) b; (7) c; (8) j; (9) f; (10) g.

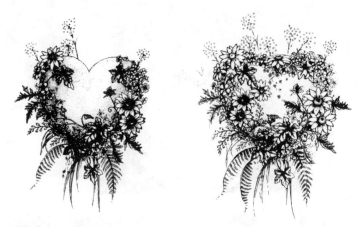

HEARTS WITH DICE,
or, Dice with Hearts

Sometimes called "hearts due," the game of hearts is designed for two or more players using six ordinary dice. Dice marked with letters spelling "HEARTS" may also be used, although this is now uncommon.

After preliminary rolls to select the first shooter (usually simply the highest scorer), the players each roll the six dice once and tally up their scores. Points are awarded as follows:

1 (H) - 5 points

1,2 (H,E) - 10 points

1,2,3 (H,E,A) - 15 points

1,2,3,4 (H,E,A,R) - 20 points

1,2,3,4,5 (H,E,A,R,T) - 25 points

1,2,3,4,5,6, (H,E,A,R,T,S) - 35 points

Play may be limited to one round, or extended to any number of rounds previously agreed upon. The winner may be either the highest scorer or the first to reach a set total, whichever the players prefer.

When a double (two dice showing the same value) or triple appears in a throw, only one will count. If, however, a player throws three 1's (or H's), he looses all points and must start over.

"And the heart that is soonest awake
  to the flowers
Is always the first to be touch'd
  by the thorns."

—Thomas Moore

(Answer to puzzle on page 47)

37

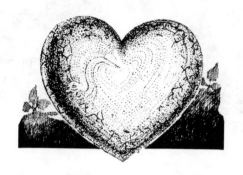

HEART'S COMPASS

Dante Gabriel Rossetti

Sometimes thou seem'st not as thyself alone,
But as the meaning of all things that are;
A breathless wonder, shadowing forth afar
Some heavenly solstice hushed and halcyon,
Whose unstirred lips are music's visible tone,
Whose eyes the sun-gate of the soul unbar,
Being of its furthest fires oracular—
The evident heart of all life sown and mown.

Even such love is; and is not thy name Love?
Yea, but thy hand the Love-god rends apart
All gathering clouds of Night's ambiguous art,
Flings them far down, and sets thine eyes above;
And simply, as some gage of flower or glove,
Stakes with a smile the world against thy heart.

Starling's Law of the Heart

No, it's not a bird's-eye view, but a biophysical principle stating that "the energy of contraction is proportional to the initial length of the cardiac muscle fiber." This means that the more the cardiac muscle fibers are stretched before the onset of contraction, the greater will be the force of that contraction. Thus Ernest Henry Starling, F.R.S. (1866—1927) demonstrated the mechanism by which the heart is automatically able to increase the energy of each contraction in proportion to the mechanical demand made upon it.

HEORTE, HERTE, HEART

The monumental *Oxford English Dictionary* covers the origins, meanings, and uses of the vocabulary of the English language. Along with definitions, the OED records the earliest known context in which each word entered our language as it was evolving from Anglo-Saxon to modern English over the course of roughly nine centuries.

For heart, the OED supplies 54 definitions (taking up 13 columns of type) and illustrates the first known use, as well as later uses, of the word in each of its meanings. The first recorded instance of the word heart—*heorte*, that is—in Old English dates back to 825 A.D.; the word is used to denote the center of the body's vital functions. The earliest documented use of heorte as an organ of the body is from the year 1000 A.D.

During the Middle English period (the twelfth through fifteenth centuries), radical linguistic changes were caused by political, social, religious, and literary influences. In this period, the word appears variously as *he(o)rt*, *herte*, and *hart*, and its expanded scope of meanings begins to become evident. The development of printing in the sixteenth century was the most important factor directing the stabilization of our ancestral language into modern English. From this time on, the form *heart* is encountered widely and in most of the senses common today.

"The Greek physiology did not divide the Self by the polarity of 'brain' and 'heart' as popular fantasies distinguish these organs of rational thinking and sympathetic feelings. In the Greek concept of the Self the brain was not valued as highly as by primitive headhunters and modern neurologists.... The intellectual capacity of man was thought to be located in the heart. The internals, and especially the heart, were considered as the undivided incarnation of man's intellectual and emotional qualities. This may be the expression of a most primitive concept of the Self. It is noteworthy that the Egyptian deities are represented with animal heads and human bodies, while in the Greek fantasies the personifications of instinctual drives appear as human above the diaphragm, as animal below it."

—Theodore Thass-Thienemann

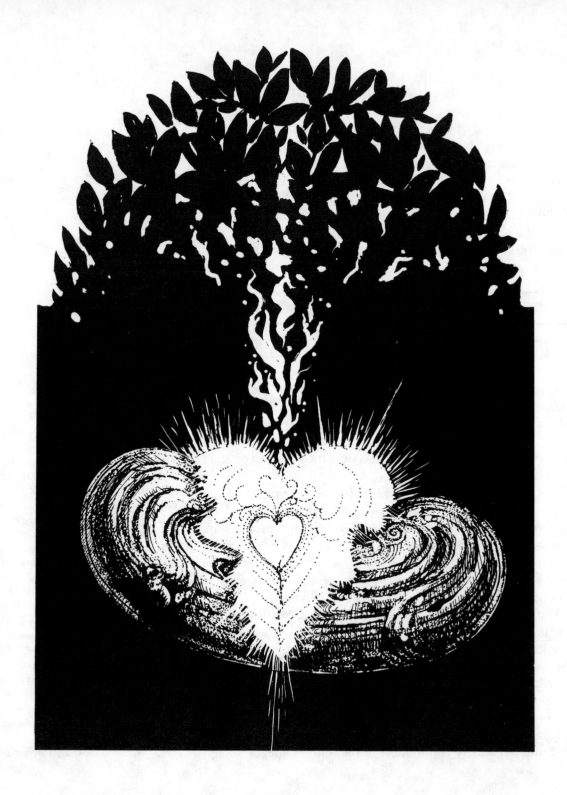

The Heart in the Cup of Gold

retold by Richard E. Nicholls

Tancred, the ruler of Salerno, was a wise and humane ruler, and his memory would be honored today, were it not that in his old age his hands became soiled by the blood of lovers (including that of the person he most loved in the world).

He had but one child, a daughter, and never did father love child more. Nor ever was child more devoted to her father. Indeed, his affection for his daughter was so great that he would become unsettled whenever she was out of his sight. For this reason, he constantly postponed any marriage agreement, finding any number of objections to suitors for his daughter's hand. But at length he was forced to consent to a marriage between his daughter and the son of the Duke of Capua. Even this, though, eventually worked out to the father's satisfaction, for his son-in-law died quite suddenly and his widowed daughter returned to her father's palace.

His daughter, whose name was Ghismonda, was a beautiful woman, a model of perfection in both form and features. She was quietly disposed, and possessed of a fine mind. Perceiving that her father's affection for her was so great that he would never allow her to remarry, and feeling that it would be immodest of her to make such a request (but being nonetheless desirous of male companionship), she decided that if she could she would secure for herself a man as lover and friend.

Her father's court saw a constant coming and going of brave Gentlemen (and others of inferior quality), and she carefully observed their carriage and demeanor. Of all she saw, one especially impressed her, a servant to her father, named Guiscardo, not noble by descent, but possessing the innate nobility of those who are virtuous. None other pleased her as the thought of Guiscardo did, and secretly she fell in love.

Guiscardo, though poor, was no insensitive lout, and he soon realized the meaning of the way in which she gazed upon him. And he, in turn, fell rapidly, deeply in love with her. She desired nothing more than to be alone with him, yet she knew she could not dare to take anyone into her heart's confidence. So she devised a cunning scheme to satisfy her desire (which grew ever more intense). She wrote a letter, explaining how their tryst could be brought about, and placed it in the joint of a hollow

41

The Heart in the Cup of Gold

cane. Then, in a jesting manner she threw it to Guiscardo, saying, "Let your man make use of this, in place of a bellows, when he comes to make a fire in your chamber." Guiscardo took up the cane, reflecting that she would not have given it to him, nor spoken such words, were there not some plan behind it. Examining the cane, he discovered the message hidden in it. And after he had read what was written therein, he was the most joyful of men, and fell to following all those instructions contained in the letter, so that he might meet with the mistress of his heart. In a corner of the palace, it being sited on a hill, there was a cave, hollowed out of the earth, and illuminated by a small opening. A secret stairway, sealed by a strong door, led from the lady's apartment down to the cave. The cave, and the door, were largely forgotten, and the entrance to the cave was overgrown. It could be reached only by someone being lowered down on a rope. Guiscardo provided himself with a rope ladder, and worked to enlarge the opening into the cave. Ghismonda spent several days carefully forcing open the rusty door to the stairway.

Guiscardo wrapped himself in a leather cloak, to avoid being scratched by brambles, and at night lowered himself into the cave. The next morning, on the excuse of being very tired, Ghismonda sent away her serving women, and retired alone to her chambers. Then with hurried step she went down into the cave, and found there her amorous friend. Ascending into the lady's chambers, they spent the better part of the day in the ways known to lovers. When at last they had to part, Guiscardo went down into the cave, and Ghismonda made fast the door behind him. Guiscardo used his rope ladder to climb out, being careful to cover the entrance of the cave behind him.

Fortune, envious of the pleasures and secrets of lovers, soon brought grief to the lovers.

Tancred was in the habit of visiting his adored daughter's chambers to talk with her. Going in one day, and finding her absent, he soon became drowsy. Lying down on a low stool at the foot of his daughter's bed, he drew the curtains about him (so that he was entirely disguised) and fell asleep. Soon after, Ghismonda came in, locking the door behind her. As that time had been appointed for a meeting with her beloved, she drew open the door to the cave, and Guiscardo entered. They did as they were wont to do, taking their delight, and the prince awakened at the sound of voices. He was confounded by what he heard and saw and was overcome with fierce grief. He formulated a plan for revenge, and for this end he remained silent, fighting back the desire to make an outcry.

The two lovers remained in each others' arms a long time. When they arose, and took tender farewell of each other, Guiscardo went back down into the cave, and Ghismonda unlocked the door and went back to her ladies. Although an old man, and none too sprightly, Tancred climbed out of a window in the room, and lowered himself down into the garden. That night, by his orders, Guiscardo was arrested as he climbed out of the cave wrapped in his leather coat. He had Guiscardo brought before him, and upbraided him for the base way in which he had repaid the prince's friendship and aid. Guiscardo hung his head, and would only answer:

"Love is more powerful than you or I."

Guiscardo was confined, and the next day Tancred went to his daughter's quarters, where he confronted her with his discovery. As he talked he cried. "Ghismonda, I have always believed that you were the most virtuous of women, and my belief in you could never have been shaken by even the worst reports. Nor could I ever imagine that you would allow any man but your husband such liberties. You cannot imagine the heartbreak I feel, having learned of your corrupt behavior. Yet if you must indulge in such weaknesses, why could you not at least have chosen a man of your own station, and not some bootless lout, some hanger-on of courts, dependent on the scraps thrown to him. I know how to proceed with him, but I confess I know not how to treat you. My mind is in a turmoil. You have murdered the love I felt for you, and kindled in me a just indignation that I should be treated so. While nature, in its guise of paternal love, pleads pardon for you, yet justice demands punishment. To determine my course, I tell you now to speak, and say what you can for yourself."

Having spoken, he hung down his head and wept. Ghismonda, though near to shrieking with grief at the certain fate of her lover, yet showed a marvelous strength (as love does sometimes give) and determined that she would not outlive Guiscardo. This decision gave her a certain serenity, and she faced her father unafraid. Thus she spoke:

The Heart
in the Cup of Gold

The Heart
in the Cup of Gold

"Tancred, I will neither deny what has been said, nor beg forgiveness. The former would not avail, and I scorn the latter. It is true that I have loved (and do love) Guiscardo. As long as I live—and I know that will not be long—I will love him. And if love survives death, I will love him then. I was not drawn to this love by any weakness, but by your refusal to allow me to remarry, and by all his noble graces. You should remember that your daughter is made of flesh and blood, and possesses the normal needs of youth for love and companionship. I could not resist the desires of the flesh, nor should I have to. And as I yielded to them, I fell in love.

"I did not choose Guiscardo on a fancy, as many women select their lovers, but was drawn to him by his character. And I believe that he who lives virtuously is the truest sort of noble, and those that live basely, no matter their parentage, can never be anything but base. Therefore, if a man lives nobly, no matter what his parentage, he can be called other than noble only by those who are blind to what nobility truly is. Consider your nobles, examine their behavior and their bearing and then compare them to Guiscardo. If you would judge without prejudice, you would have to agree that of all of them Guiscardo is most noble, and all the rest little better than peasants. Indeed, who has praised him more for his valiant deeds than you? You may say that he is a poor man. You may say that he was not born into the nobility. But you cannot deny that he possesses all those qualities that make a man truly noble, and for which he should be praised.

"I care not what you do to me. I will not beg forgiveness for something I consider not to have been wrong, as I have only followed the dictates of my heart. Indeed, I tell you now that if you do not do to me what you do to Guiscardo, I shall inflict it on myself with my own hands.

"Go, then, and weep, and if you would cruelly kill him, favor me by killing me with the same stroke."

Tancred left his daughter, much amazed by her resolute behavior. But he did not believe she could be so determined as to kill herself, and he decided to cool her ardor by punishing her in other ways.

That night he had Guiscardo strangled, and the lover's heart was cut out and carried to Tancred. Next day he had it placed in a gold cup, and sent it to his daughter. She, meanwhile, fearing the

44

worst, had secretly obtained herbs and roots of a poisonous nature, and distilled from them a fatal draught. When she was presented with the cup, and saw the heart within, she knew that Guiscardo was dead, and that she must follow.

She spoke tenderly to the heart, letting her tears fall upon it. Again and again she kissed her lover's heart. Her women did not know whose heart it was, and were astonished at Ghismonda's tears, sighs, and words. They were all so moved by the sight that they too broke into lamentations. Then Ghismonda took up the bottle containing the poison and poured it into the golden cup holding the heart, and fearlessly drank the draught. Having drained the cup, she lay down upon her bed, arranged her body modestly, and laying the heart of her lover upon her heart, silently waited for death to release her.

Tancred, being sent for, came at once and realized what his daughter had done. Then did he weep so uncontrollably that he could not utter a word. His daughter asked simply that she and Guiscardo be buried together. Then, knowing that her end had come, she clutched her lover's heart to her, and said simply, "God be with you, and let me go."

Tancred was overcome with the results of his wrath. He lived for but a short time, and that time filled with grief.

As Ghismonda had wished, the lovers were buried together and all Salerno mourned their tragedy.

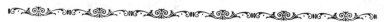

In the desert
I saw a creature, naked, bestial,
Who, squatting upon the ground,
Held his heart in his hands
And ate of it.
I said, "Is it good, friend?"
"It is bitter—bitter," he answered;
"But I like it
"Because it is bitter,
"And because it is my heart."

THE HEART
by Stephen Crane

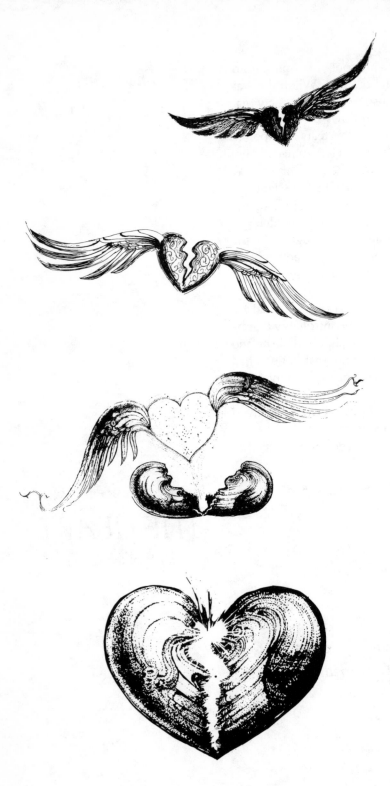

DOWN

1 Flier Amelia
2 Cast aspersions on
3 —— Marquette
4 Lively in spite of age
5 Miss Tallchief et al.
6 Upright
7 "Wake Up and ——"
8 Depot: Abbr.
9 Completely
10 Center of an escutcheon
11 Gaelic
12 Butterfly and hair
13 Part of C.B.S.: Abbr.
21 Finished
23 Defeat soundly
25 Prefixes for heart cavities
26 Words of affection
27 Apportion
28 Swedish port
29 Salisbury ——
30 Aftermath of overeating
31 Uncanny
32 Apollo's birthplace
34 Do, re, mi, fa, ——, ti
37 Memorize
38 Timorous
40 Portico
41 Biblical wall tower
43 Sorrow
44 Lear's daughter et al.
46 Hindu deity and others
47 Spanish uncles
48 Icelandic writing
49 Cad
50 Superman's Lois
51 Cordially
52 Common Latin verb
53 Of stock, in old Ireland
56 Aunt or uncle: Abbr.

CROSS MY HEART

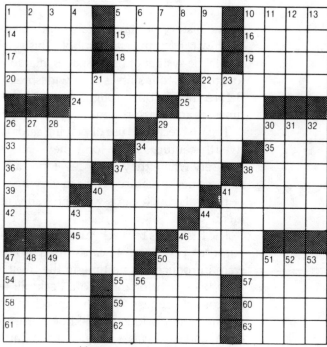

(Answer to puzzle will be found on page 37.)

ACROSS

1 Catch sight of
5 "Act One" author
10 Gives courage to
14 Gambler, in old Rome
15 Miss Loos
16 Victim
17 N.Z. bird
18 French historian
19 Kilns
20 Pitiable
22 Most arid
24 Spur

25 "Unto us —— is given"
26 Coneys
29 Dauntless
33 Gladden
34 Walk pompously
35 Busy one
36 Extremely generous
37 Trompe —— (visual deception
38 Roll up, as a flag
39 Type of novel: Abbr.
40 Burmese rices
41 Mr. Lanza
42 Frank discussion

44 French queens
45 Adriatic wind
46 Writer O'Casey
47 Iran's capital
50 Carefree
54 French thought
55 Cape Verde island
57 "The —— Lonely Hunter"
58 Concert halls
59 City of China
60 Otherwise
61 Polio pioneer
62 Unfeeling
63 Colorist

HEARTS & PLAYING CARDS

The history of playing cards aptly demonstrates the fact that the heart is a universal symbol. This is less odd than it sounds. While the system of using spades, diamonds, clubs, and hearts to identify the four suits is now widespread, it was not always so. Before these won through, a remarkably diverse—and sometimes bizarre—assortment of symbols were featured.

The first recorded use of playing cards was in the Orient, in the twelfth century. How long they had previously existed and precisely where they were developed are unknown. Very early Chinese decks featured coins in varying numbers to denote each of the suits. Such cards were probably used simply for amusement.

The first cards to reach Europe had an ostensibly more serious purpose. These "tarot" cards, used as an aid in fortune-telling, were introduced some time in the twelfth century. There may have been fifty or more to a deck, all featuring hand-painted allegorical scenes. Wealthy merchants and members of the nobility commissioned well-known artists to paint tarot decks for them, and each was a unique work of art. Indeed, because each deck had to be painted by hand, only the wealthy could afford them. The introduction of the printing press gradually changed all that. By the sixteenth century, cards were a familiar sight, widely available and very popular.

And they were no longer simply for divination or for show. They had become the basis of a number of games. Just when and how this happened is unclear, although there is evidence to show that as early as the fourteenth century many games using cards were already widely known. Indeed, even though they were very expensive, the market for cards was large enough for England and some of the city-states of Italy to enforce embargoes forbidding importers from bringing in the handsome decks produced in Germany because native cardmakers were being driven out of business by the competition.

Because each cardmaker favored his own symbols and ideas, literally hundreds were used to represent the four suits—everything from mythological beasts to wild animals to acorns. Even the number of cards in a deck fluctuated. The advent of the printing press helped to bring a certain uniformity to the field. Playing cards became more and more standarized, with fewer individual quirks.

It was left to a French knight to bring even more uniformity to the field when, in the sixteenth century, he invented the "modern" deck of cards in which the four suits are represented by hearts, diamonds (or squares), clovers, and pikeheads. The heart had been used as early as the fourteenth century as a symbol for one of the suits. That it should have endured is not surprising—it is a universal symbol, immediately recognizable, and its simplicity lends itself well to the design of a deck of cards.

The English enthusiastically adopted the French deck and in the process further simplified the symbols into today's spades, hearts, diamonds, and clubs. Cards quickly became a very popular means of entertainment among all levels of society. This is testified to by the fact that as early as 1633 some miscreant New England Puritans were caught in a game of cards and fined the stiff sum of two pounds each for their moral lapse. That cards should be used even by the isolationist Puritans hidden away in North America shows how rapidly those first curious tarot decks had evolved from a prop for prophets of the future into something quite different.

"The heart, ready furnished with its proper organs of motion, like a kind of internal creature, existed before the body. The first to be formed, nature willed that it should afterwards fashion, nourish, preserve, complete the entire animal, as its work and dwelling-place: and as the prince in a kingdom, in whose hands lie the chief and highest authority, rules over all, the heart is the source and foundation from which all power is derived, on which all power depends in the animal body."—William Harvey

---

The human heart is like a millstone in a mill; when you put wheat under it, it turns and grinds, and bruises the wheat into flour; if you put no wheat in it, it still grinds on; but then it is itself it grinds, and slowly wears away.
—Martin Luther

Annual Hearty Fairs

Heart of Florida Folk Festival
  (Dade City, Fla., Feb.-March)
Heart of The Hills Days
  (Hill City, S.D., mid-July)
Heart O'Texas Fair
  (Waco, Tex., October)
Heart of the Ozarks Fair
  (West Plains, Mo., mid-June)

BROADWAY HEARTS

Select the musical show in which each of the following heart songs appears.

1. *A Dream Is a Wish Your Heart Makes.* (a) Frankie and Johnny; (b) A Tree Grows in Brooklyn; (c) Disneyland; (d) The Fantasticks.

2. *Heart ("You Gotta Have Heart").* (a) Can-Can; (b) Plain and Fancy; (c) Seventeen; (d) Damn Yankees.

3. *My Heart Belongs to Daddy.* (a) Leave It to Me; (b) Fiddler on the Roof; (c) Sweethearts; (d) L'il Abner.

4. *My Heart is Full of You.* (a) All For Love; (b) Most Happy Fella; (c) Fanny; (d) Always in My Heart.

5. *My Heart Stood Still.* (a) Connecticut Yankees; (b) Oklahoma; (c) Three Coins in a Fountain; (d) You're a Sweetheart.

6. *Raining in My Heart.* (a) My Fair Lady; (b) Carefree Heart; (c) The Student Prince; (d) Dames at Sea.

7. *Two Hearts Are Better Than One.* (a) Merry Widow; (b) Centennial Summer; (c) South Pacific; (d) The World of Charles Aznavour.

8. *Way To a Man's Heart.* (a) L'il Abner; (b) Carnival; (c) One Hour With You; (d) High Society.

9. *With a Song in My Heart.* (a) The Blossom; (b) Seventeen; (c) Spring Is Here; (d) Carefree Heart.

10. *Zing! Went the Strings of My Heart.* (a) Conversation Piece; (b) How To Succeed in Business Without Really Trying; (c) Queen High; (d) Thumbs Up.

The heart-leaved cucumber tree, a southern U.S. magnolia, takes its name from the cordiform shape of its leaves. It has been observed that people desire this tree as much for its symmetrical form as for the beauty of its flowers and its luxuriant foliage.

ANSWERS: (1) c; (2) d; (3) a; (4) b; (5) a; (6) d; (7) b; (8) a; (9) c; (10) d.

50

THE NUTRITIOUS HEART

Type of Heart	Measure or Quantity	Protein (grams)	Calories
Beef:			
Lean, raw	1 lb.	77.6	490
Lean, braised	4 oz.	35.5	213
Lean, braised, chopped or diced	1 cup (5.1 oz.)	45.4	273
Lean with visible fat, raw	1 lb.	69.9	1148
Lean with visible fat, braised	4 oz.	29.3	422
Calf, raw	1 lb.	68.0	562
Calf, braised	4 oz.	31.5	236
Chicken, raw	1 lb.	84.4	608
Chicken, simmered	1 heart (5 grams)	1.3	9
Chicken, simmered, chopped, or diced	1 cup (5.1 oz.)	36.7	251
Hog, raw	1 lb.	76.2	513
Hog, braised	4 oz.	34.9	221
Lamb, raw	1 lb.	76.2	735
Lamb, braised	4 oz.	33.5	295
Turkey, raw	1 lb.	73.5	776
Turkey, simmered	4 oz.	25.6	245
Turkey, simmered, chopped, or diced	1 cup (5.1 oz.)	32.8	313

(USDA): United States Department of Agriculture

"... an organ that grows hard quicker in riches than an egg boiling in water."
—Ludwig Boerne

"The heart may be compared to a wurst: no one can tell exactly what's inside."—Jewish saying

"When a butcher tells you his heart bleeds for his country, he has, in fact, no uneasy feeling."
—Samuel Johnson

MILESTONES in the STUDY of the HEART

1628 **Circulation of the Blood** through the body was described by William Harvey, an English physician.

1706 **The Structure of the Left Ventricle and Distribution of Coronary Vessels** were described by Raymond de Vieussens, a French anatomy professor.

1733 **Blood Pressure** was measured by Stephen Hales, an English clergyman and scientist.

1785 **Digitalis,** in the form of foxglove leaves, was introduced by William Withering, English physician.

1816 **The Stethoscope** was invented by Rene T.H. Laennec, a French physician.

1893 **The Atrioventricular Bundle,** a muscle bundle connecting the right atrium with the ventricles of the heart, was discovered by Wilhelm His, Jr., a Swiss anatomist. It is also called the *bundle of His.*

1903 **The Electrocardiograph,** for showing the heart's electrical activity, was developed by Willem Einthoven, a Dutch physiologist.

1904 **The Effect of Rheumatic Fever** on the heart was described by Ludwig Aschoff, a German pathologist.

1908 **Congential Heart Disease** was described and classified by Maude Abbott, a Canadian physician.

1912 **First Diagnosis of Coronary Thrombosis** and description of heart disease resulting from hardening of the arteries were made by James B. Herrick, an American cardiologist.

1930 **Modern Method of Electrocardiology** was developed by Frank N. Wilson, an American physician.

1944 **First Surgery for Blue Babies** was performed by Alfred Blalock, an American surgeon, and Helen B. Taussig, an American cardiologist.

1948 **First Successful Operations** for rheumatic heart disease were performed independently by Charles P. Bailey and Dwight E. Harken, American surgeons.

1951 **Plastic Ball Valve** for a leaky aortic (semilunar) valve was developed by Charles Hufnagel, an American surgeon.

1952 **Open Heart Surgery** was first successfully performed by F. John Lewis, an American surgeon. He used ice to lower body temperature and slow circulation so the heart remained dry during surgery.

1953 **Mechanical Heart and Blood Purifier** was used successfully for the first time by John H. Gibbon, an American surgeon.

1954 **Human Cross-Circulation,** permitting a second person's heart and lungs to pump blood of a person under surgery, was developed by C. Walton Lillehei, an American surgeon.

1961 **External Cardiac Massage,** to restart a stopped heart without surgery, was introduced by J.R. Jude, an American cardiologist, and his associates.

1962 **Cardioversion,** a method of correcting fibrillation and irregular heart beat by electric shock, was introduced by B. Lown, an American cardiologist.

1965 **Assisting Hearts,** mechanical devices to help a diseased or overworked left ventricle, were first successfully implanted by Michael E. De Bakey, and by Adrian Kantrowitz, American surgeons.

1967 **First Transplant** of a whole heart from one person to another was performed by a surgical team headed by Christiaan Barnard of South Africa.

1974 **First Implantation** of a donor heart without removing the patient's own heart was performed by a surgical team headed by Christiaan Barnard.

From *The World Book Encyclopedia,* © 1978 World Book-Childcraft International, Inc.

The heart transplant to survive the longest is Emmanuel Vitria, 58, of Marseilles, France. Since he received his new heart 9½ years ago, Vitria has taken 20,000 pills and had 11,000 injections. The side effects of these drugs have caused the tissue in his spinal column to become compressed, making him 7 inches shorter.

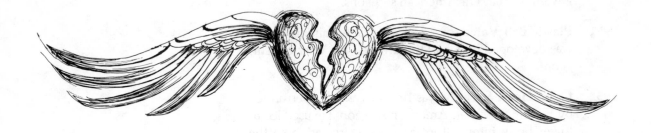

The Heart of Dionysus

Dionysus is remembered today as the Greek god of wine and ecstasy. In fact, the beliefs centering on Dionysus were considerably more complex than that. He was also worshipped as a certain proof of the resurrection and survival of the soul after death. Central to this belief were tales explaining Dionysus' death and remarkable resurrection. And in many of these tales, the heart of Dionysus had a central place.

The tales describing Dionysus' death differ in many particulars. But all of them agree on the manner of his death: he was torn to pieces, the pieces then being either widely scattered or consumed by the supernatural creatures that had murdered him. In some versions, Dionysus' mother, the goddess Semele, succeeded in gathering all the pieces of his body together, and in reanimating them. In the versions of Dionysus' martyrdom in which his body is consumed by his enemies, only his heart is preserved from the appetites of his foes. Then Zeus, the most powerful of all the Greek gods, either swallows the heart and then begets Dionysus again upon Semele, or he causes the heart to be reduced to a powder, which is mixed in a potion and given to Semele. And from the potion she again conceives and gives birth to Dionysus.

Belief in the immortality of the soul was an important tenet of the Dionysian faith. The heart, as the symbol of the core of each human personality, representative of the soul, understandably became the focus of the tales concerning this belief.

"Bear, O my heart; thou has borne a yet harder thing."—Homer

"The pleasures of the intellect are permanent, the pleasures of the heart are transitory."
—Henry David Thoreau

How Coyote Stole God's Heart

The Yuman Indians of California tell a story of how their god died, poisoned by an evil and envious being. The people mourned bitterly. Now that they had lost their god, death had finally come among them.

Now Coyote wanted the heart of the god because he believed it would make him strong. He tried every trick his wily brain could think of to steal the heart away, but the people always beat him back. However, during the god's cremation ceremony, just as the body was about to be consumed by the flames, Coyote made a great leap onto the funeral pyre, snatched the heart, and ran away with it.

One tribe of California Indians, the Juaneno, had a mourning ritual in which this folk tale figured. Since the "heart" of a dead person was understood to be the soul, when anyone died a figure acting as the *ano* (Coyote) would cut a piece of flesh from the dead person's shoulder and eat it. In this ritual, the flesh represented the heart, and by eating it the soul was released. It could then leave the body and ascend to the sky, where it became a star.

The Bower of Love

"One will grant the heart a modicum of history," writes Richard Selzer. "Ancient man slew his enemy, then fell upon the corpse to cut out his heart, which he ate with gusto, for it was well understood that to devour the slain enemy's heart was to take upon oneself the strength, valor and skill of the vanquished. It was not the livers or brains or entrails of saints that were lifted from the body in sublimest autopsy, it was the heart, thus snipped and cradled into worshipful palms, then soaked in wine and herbs and set into silver reliquaries for the veneration of the faithful. It follows quite naturally that Love should choose such an organ for its bower. In the absence of Love, the canker gnaws it; when Love blooms therein, the heart dances and *tremor cordis* is upon one."

My heart leaps up when I behold
  A rainbow in the sky:
So was it when my life began;
So is it now I am a man;
So be it when I shall grow old,
  Or let me die!
The Child is father of the Man;
And I could wish my days to be
Bound each to each by natural piety.

—William Wordsworth

DR. JOHNSON DEFINES
HEART

Dr. Samuel Johnson's *Dictionary of the English Language* (1755), the first authoritative, comprehensive work of its kind in English, gives twenty-one meanings or usages for the term heart, to which list the pioneering lexicographer adds a couple dozen popular compound heart terms.

HEART. (1) The muscle which, by its contraction and dilation, propels the blood through the course of circulation, and is therefore considered as the source of vital motion. (2) It is supposed in popular language to be the seat sometimes of courage, sometimes of affection, sometimes of honesty, or baseness. (3) The chief part; the vital part; the vigorous or efficacious part. (4) The inner part of any thing. (5) Person, character; used with respect to courage or kindness. (6) Courage, spirit. (7) Seat of love. (8) Affection; inclination. (9) Memory. (10) Good-will; ardour or zeal. To take to heart any thing, is to be zealous or solicitous or ardent about it. (11) Passion; anxiety; concern. (12) Secret thoughts; recesses of the mind. (13) Disposition of mind. (14) The heart is considered as the seat of tenderness; a hard heart therefore is cruelty. (15) To find in the heart; to be not wholly averse. (16) Secret meaning; hidden intention. (17) Conscience; sense of good or ill. (18) Strength; power; vigour; efficacy. (19) Utmost degree. (20) Life. For my heart seems sometimes to signify, if life was at stake; and sometimes for tenderness. (21) It is much used in composition for mind, or affection.

HEART-ACHE. Sorrow; pang; anguish of mind.
HEART-BREAK. Overpowering sorrow.
HEART-BREAKER. A cant name for a woman's curls, supposed to break the heart of all her lovers.

Phrases of the Heart

to have a hard heart
a change of heart
out of heart
to eat one's heart out
to make one's heart leap
heavy at heart
near to one's heart
heart-to-heart talk
to pluck up heart
to have at heart
to lose heart
with all one's heart
hearts of oak
to be down in the heart
to set one's heart at rest
to put in good heart
to win someone's heart
to put one's heart into
hale and hearty
to be of good heart
half-hearted
sick at heart
to wear one's heart on one's sleeve
to pluck out the heart of the mystery
to have one's heart in one's mouth
to have a soft place in the heart for

HEART-BREAKING   Overpowering with sorrow; over-
    powering grief.
HEART-BURNED.   Having the heart inflamed.
HEART-BURNING.   1. Pain at the stomach, commonly
    from an acrid humour.   2. Discontent; secret enmity.
HEART-DEAR.   Sincerely beloved.
HEART-EASE.   Quiet; tranquility.
HEARTS-EASE.   A plant.
HEART-FELT.   Felt in the conscience.
HEART-PEAS.   A plant with round seeds in form of peas,
    of black colour, having the figure of a heart of a white
    colour upon each.
HEART-QUELLING.   Conquering the affection.
HEART-RENDING.   Killing with anguish.
HEART-ROBBING.   Depriving of thought.
HEART-SICK.   1. Pained in mind.   2. Mortally ill; hurt
    in the heart.
HEART-SORE.   That which pains the mind.
HEART-STRING.   The tendons or nerves supposed to
    brace and sustain the heart.
HEART-STRUCK.   1. Driven to the heart; infixed for
    ever in the mind.   2. Shocked with fear or dismay.
HEART-SWELLING.   Rankling in the mind.
HEART-WHOLE.   1. With the affections yet unfixed.
    2. With the vitals yet unimpaired.
HEART-WOUNDING.   Filling with grief.
HEARTED.   It is only used in composition, as, hard
    hearted.
To HEARTEN.   1. To encourage; to animate; to stir up.
    2. To meliorate or renovate with manure.
HEART-WOUNDED.   Filled with passion of love or grief.

to keep heart
to learn by heart
to take heart
chicken-hearted
have a heart
to break one's heart
down-hearted
with one's whole heart
after one's heart
to lose one's heart
to take to heart
next to the heart
to be the heart and soul of
heart-rending
to touch the heart of
whole-hearted
to find in one's heart to
to search the heart
heart-felt
to have a soft heart
a heart of gold
to one's heart's content
heart of stone
soft-hearted
with heart and hand
to have the heart to
to do one's heart good
to give heart to
bless your heart
to take heart of grace
heart-sick
to give one's heart
heart-whole
in one's heart of hearts
with half a heart
to set one's heart on
to have one's heart in the right place
from the bottom of the heart
to warm the cockles of the heart

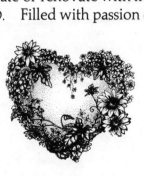

"No heart attack is ever really 'sudden.' It may seem that way to the patient and family members, but coronary disease has in all likelihood been building over the years, helped along by the patient who has ignored the risk factors and failed to heed the early warning signals." —*AHA*

THE AMERICAN HEART ASSOCIATION
National Center
7320 Greenville Ave.
Dallas, Texas 75231

The American Heart Association is a nonprofit, nationwide network composed of some 55 affiliate organizations which all work to reduce the crippling and fatal results of heart and blood vessel diseases. Since 1949, the AHA has spent a quarter of a billion dollars on research into the causes, treatment, and prevention of heart disease. Some of the results of this long-term research include the development of the pacemaker and artificial heart valves, the invention of the heart-lung machine, and the implementation of new drugs and surgical techniques.

The AHA sponsors community programs all across the country. These serve to identify potential heart disease victims, diagnose people suffering from high blood pressure, train both laymen and medical personnel in emergency cardiac care techniques such as CPR (cardiopulmonary resuscitation), and provide rehabilitation for those who have suffered heart attacks and strokes. In addition, the AHA sponsors programs to keep physicians up to date on the most recent research on heart disease as well as the newest methods for treating heart and blood vessel diseases.

The Association is able to carry out its programs only because of the money donated every year by the American public. In 1976, heart associations raised some 67 million dollars to finance AHA projects. Much of this money was spent in the local areas in which it was collected.

Newsweek magazine (May 8, 1978) reported that John Wayne received the mitral valve of a pig's heart to replace a defective valve in his heart. Convalescing from open-heart surgery, Wayne remarked, "I feel like a new man. When I wake up in the morning and it's raining, I feel like rolling in the mud."

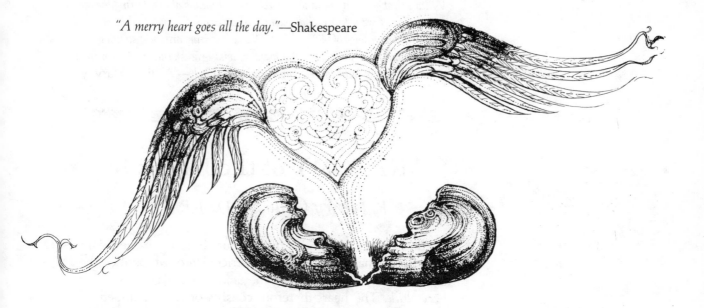

"A merry heart goes all the day."—Shakespeare

BIG-HEARTED HONORS

Among almost a dozen awards regularly given by the American Heart Association are the following:

The *Gold Heart Award* is presented annually to an individual in recognition of distinguished service to the association and a notable contribution to the national heart program.

The *Heart and Torch Award* honors prominent persons in the field of radio, television, motion pictures, and other mass media who have distinguished themselves in noteworthy service to the Heart Fund campaign.

The *Heart of the Year Award* is given annually to a distinguished American in recognition of personal achievement, faith, and courage in meeting the challenge of heart disease.

The Purple Heart is a U.S. military decoration awarded to any member of the armed forces who has been wounded in action.

When I first gave my mind to vivisection, as a means of discovering the motions and uses of the heart, and sought to discover these from actual inspection, and not from writings of others, I found the task so truly arduous, so full of difficulties, that I was almost tempted to think, with Fracastorius, that the motion of the heart was only to be comprehended by God. —William Harvey

ANATOMY of the HEART

by *Henry Gray*, M.D., F.R.S.

According to Aristotle, the hearts of horses and some breeds of oxen contained a bone that provided support for the organ.

The Egyptian Book of the Dead devotes six chapters to the heart, the only visceral organ to be retained when a body was mummified. It was crucial that the heart accompany the deceased to the netherworld since his fate would be decided when Osiris weighed the heart in his judgement hall.

The Egyptians believed that blood vessels carried and filtered not only blood but human waste. It was thus possible for such wastes to be carried to the heart and damage it.

The human heart is divided by a septum into two halves, right and left, each half being further constricted into two cavities, the upper of the two being termed the *auricle* [atrium] and the lower the *ventricle*. The heart therefore consists of four chambers or cavities, two forming the right half, the right auricle and right ventricle, and two the left half, the left auricle and left ventricle. The right half of the heart contains venous or impure blood; the left, arterial or pure blood. From the cavity of the left ventricle the pure blood is carried into a large artery, the *aorta*, through the numerous branches of which it is distributed to all parts of the body, with the exception of the lungs. In its passage through the capillaries of the body the blood gives up to the tissues the materials necessary for their growth and nourishment, and at the same time receives from the tissues the waste products resulting from their metabolism, and in doing so becomes changed from arterial or pure blood into venous or impure blood, which is collected by the veins and through them returned to the right auricle of the heart. From this cavity the impure blood passes into the right ventricle, from which it is conveyed through the *pulmonary arteries* to the lungs. In the capillaries of the lungs it again becomes arterialized, and is then carried to the left auricle by the *pulmonary veins*. From this cavity it passes into that of the left ventricle, from which the cycle once more begins.

—from the Unabridged Running Press
Edition of Gray's Anatomy

NEVER GIVE ALL HEART

William Butler Yeats

Never give all the heart, for love
Will hardly seem worth thinking of
To passionate women if it seem
Certain, and they never dream
That it fades out from kiss to kiss;
For everything that's lovely is
But a brief, dreamy, kind of delight.
O never give the heart outright,
For they, for all smooth lips can say,
Have given their hearts up to the play.
And who could play it well enough
If deaf and dumb and blind with love?
He that made this knows all the cost,
For he gave all his heart and lost.

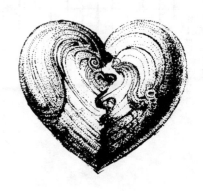

A Shakespearean Cardiograph

The graph below shows the number of times, according to the *Oxford Shakespeare Concordances*, that Shakespeare used the word heart or a heart-like word (such as heartily, heartless) in each of his plays. The plays are listed chronologically from left to right. Scholars may conclude that in some of the early plays the word heart is used often and in some it is not. The same apparently holds true for the later plays.

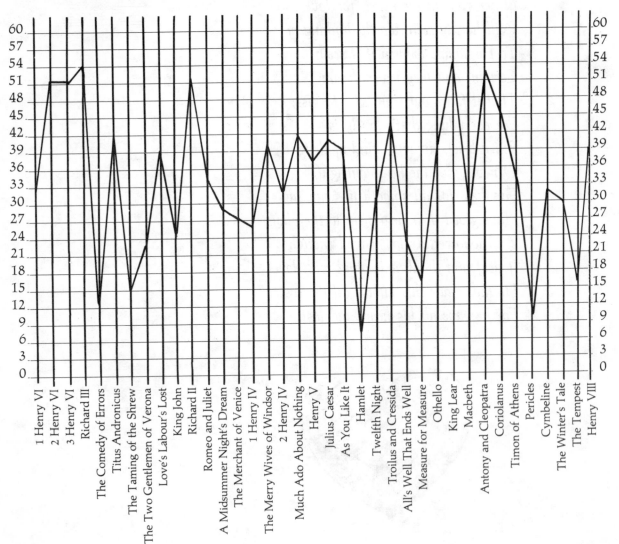

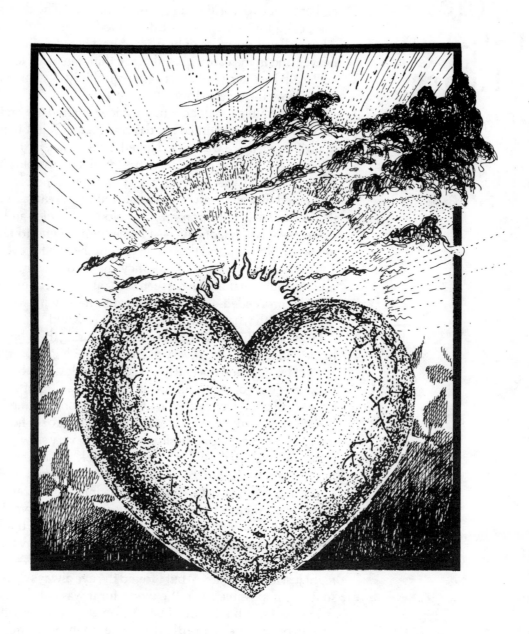

The Tell-Tale Heart

by Edgar Allen Poe

TRUE!——nervous——very, very dreadfully nervous I had been and am ! but why *will* you say that I am mad? The disease had sharpened my senses——not destroyed——not dulled them. Above all was the sense of hearing acute. I heard all things in the heaven and in the earth. I heard many things in hell. How, then, am I mad? Hearken ! and observe how healthily——how calmly I can tell you the whole story.

It is impossible to say how first the idea entered my brain; but once conceived, it haunted me day and night. Object there was none. Passion there was none. I loved the old man. He had never wronged me. He had never given me insult. For his gold I had no desire. I think it was his eye! yes, it was this! One of his eyes resembled that of a vulture——a pale blue eye, with a film over it. Whenever it fell upon me, my blood ran cold; and so by degrees——very gradually——I made up my mind to take the life of the old man, and thus rid myself of the eye for ever.

Now this is the point. You fancy me mad. Madmen know nothing. But you should have seen *me.* You should have seen how wisely I proceeded——with what caution——with what fore-sight——with what dissimulation I went to work!

I was never kinder to the old man than during the whole week before I killed him. And every night, about midnight, I turned the latch of his door and opened it——oh, so gently! And then, when I had made an opening sufficient for my head, I put in a dark lantern, all closed, closed, so that no light shone out, and then I thrust in my head. Oh, you would have laughed to see how cunningly I thrust it in! I moved it slowly——very, very slowly, so that I might not disturb the old man's sleep. It took me an hour to place my whole head within the opening so far that I could see him as he lay upon his bed. Ha!——would a madman have been so wise as this? And then, when my head was well in the room, I undid the lantern cautiously——oh, so cautiously——(for the hinges creaked)——I undid it just so much that a single thin ray fell upon the vulture eye. And this I did for seven long nights——every night just at midnight——but I found the eye always closed; and so it was impossible to do the work; for it was not the old man who vexed me, but his Evil Eye. And every morning, when the day broke, I went boldly into the chamber, and spoke courageously to him, calling him by name in a hearty tone, and inquiring how he had passed the night. So you see he would have been a very profound old man, indeed, to suspect that every night, just at twelve, I looked in upon him while he slept.

Upon the eighth night I was more than usually cautious in opening the door. A watch's minute hand moves more quickly than did mine. Never before that night had I *felt* the extent of my own powers——of my sagacity. I could scarcely contain my feelings of triumph. To think that there I was, opening the door, little by little, and he not even to dream of my secret deeds or thoughts. I fairly chuckled at the idea; and perhaps he heard me; for he moved on the bed suddenly, as if startled. Now you may think that I drew back——but no. His room was as black as pitch with the thick darkness, (for the shutters were close fastened, through fear of robbers,) and so I knew that he could not see the opening of the door, and I kept pushing it on steadily, steadily.

I had my head in, and was about to open the lantern, when my thumb slipped upon the tin fastening, and the old man sprang up in the bed, crying out——"Who's there?"

I kept quite still and said nothing. For a whole hour I did not move a muscle, and in the meantime I did not hear him lie down. He was still sitting up in the bed listening;—— just as I have done, night after night, hearkening to the death watches in the wall.

Presently I heard a slight groan, and I knew it was the groan of mortal terror. It was not a groan of pain or of grief——oh no! ——it was the low stifled sound that arises from the bottom of the soul when overcharged with awe. I knew the sound well. Many a night, just at midnight, when all the world slept, it has welled up from my own bosom, deepening, with its dreadful echo, the terrors that distracted me. I say I knew it well. I knew what the old man felt, and pitied him, although I chuckled at heart. I knew that he had been lying awake ever since the first slight noise, when he had turned in the bed. His fears had been ever since growing upon him. He had been trying to fancy them causeless, but could not. He had been saying to himself——"It is nothing but the wind in the chimney—— it is only a mouse crossing the floor," or "it is merely a cricket which has made a single chirp." Yes, he has been trying to comfort himself with these suppositions; but he had found all in vain. *All in vain;* because Death, in approaching him, had stalked with his black shadow before him, and enveloped the victim. And it was the mournful influence of the unperceived shadow that caused him to feel——although he neither saw nor

The Tell-Tale Heart

heard——to *feel* the presence of my head within the room.

When I had waited a long time, very patiently, without hearing him lie down, I resolved to open a little——a very, very little crevice in the lantern. So I opened it——you cannot imagine how stealthily, stealthily——until, at length, a single dim ray, like the thread of the spider, shot from out the crevice and full upon the vulture eye.

It was open——wide, wide open——and I grew furious as I gazed upon it. I saw it with perfect distinctness——all a dull blue, with a hideous veil over it that chilled the very marrow in my bones; but I could see nothing else of the old man's face or person: for I had directed the ray as if by instinct, precisely upon the damned spot.

And now have I not told you that what you mistake for madness is but over-acuteness of the senses?——now, I say, there came to my ears a low, dull, quick sound, such as a watch makes when enveloped in cotton. I knew *that* sound well too. It was the beating of the old man's heart. It increased my fury, as the beating of a drum stimulates the soldier into courage.

But even yet I refrained and kept still. I scarcely breathed. I held the lantern motionless. I tried how steadily I could maintain the ray upon the eye. Meantime the hellish tattoo of the heart increased. It grew quicker and quicker, and louder and louder every instant. The old man's terror *must* have been extreme! It grew louder, I say, louder every moment!——do you mark me well? I have told you that I am nervous: so I am. And now at the dead hour of the night, amid the dreadful silence of that old house, so strange a noise as this excited me to uncontrollable terror. Yet, for some minutes longer I refrained and stood still. But the beating grew louder, louder! I thought the heart must burst. And now a new anxiety seized me——the sound would be heard by a neighbor! The old man's hour had come! With a loud yell, I threw open the lantern and leaped into the room. He shrieked once——once only. In an instant I dragged him to the floor, and pulled the heavy bed over him. I then smiled gaily, to find the deed so far done. But, for many minutes, the heart beat on with a muffled sound. This, however, did not vex me; it would not be heard through the wall. At length it ceased. The old man was dead. I removed the bed and examined the corpse. Yes, he was stone, stone dead. I placed my hand upon the heart and held it there many minutes. There was no pulsation. He was stone dead. His eye would trouble me no more.

If still you think me mad, you will think so no longer when I describe the wise precautions I took for the concealment of the body. The night waned, and I worked hastily, but in silence. First of all I dismembered the corpse. I cut off the head and the arms and the legs.

I then took up three planks from the flooring of the chamber, and deposited all between the scantlings. I then replaced the boards so cleverly, so cunningly, that no human eye——not even *his*——could have detected any thing wrong. There was nothing to wash out——no stain of any kind——no blood-spot whatever. I had been too wary for that. A tub had caught all——ha! ha!

When I had made an end of these labors, it was four o'clock——still dark as midnight. As the bell sounded the hour, there came a knocking at the street door. I went down to open it with a light heart,——for what had I *now* to fear? There entered three men, who introduced themselves, with perfect suavity, as officers of the police. A shriek had been heard by a neighbor during the night; suspicion of foul play had been aroused; information had been lodged at the police office, and they (the officers) had been deputed to search the premises.

I smiled,——for *what* had I to fear? I bade the gentlemen welcome. The shriek, I said, was my own in a dream. The old man, I mentioned, was absent in the country. I took my visitors all over the house. I bade them search——search *well*. I led them, at length, to *his* chamber. I showed them his treasures, secure, undisturbed. In the enthusiasm of my confidence, I brought chairs into the room, and desired them *here* to rest from their fatigues, while I myself, in the wild audacity of my perfect triumph, placed my own seat upon the very spot beneath which reposed the corpse of the victim.

The officers were satisfied. My *manner* had convinced them. I was singularly at ease. They sat, and while I answered cheerily, they chatted familiar things. But, ere long, I felt myself getting pale and wished them gone. My head ached, and I fancied a ringing in my ears: but still they sat and still chatted. The ringing became more distinct:——it continued and became more distinct: I talked more freely to get rid of the feeling: but it continued and gained definitiveness——until, at length, I found that

The Tell-Tale Heart

The Tell-Tale Heart

the noise was *not* within my ears.

No doubt I now grew *very* pale;——but I talked more fluently, and with a heightened voice. Yet the sound increased——and what could I do? It was *a low, dull, quick sound——much such a sound as a watch makes when enveloped in cotton.* I gasped for breath——and yet the officers heard it not. I talked more quickly——more vehemently; but the noise steadily increased. I arose and argued about trifles, in a high key and with violent gesticulations, but the noise steadily increased. Why *would* they not be gone? I paced the floor to and fro with heavy strides, as if excited to fury by the observation of the men——but the noise steadily increased. Oh God! what *could* I do? I foamed——I raved——I swore! I swung the chair upon which I had been sitting, and grated it upon the boards, but the noise arose over all and continually increased. It grew louder——louder——*louder!* And still the men chatted pleasantly, and smiled. Was it possible they heard not? Almighty God!——no, no! They heard!——they suspected!——they *knew!*—— they were making a *mockery* of my horror!——this I thought, and this I think. But any thing was better than this agony! Any thing was more tolerable than this derision! I could bear those hypocritical smiles no longer! I felt that I must scream or die!——and now——again!——hark! louder! louder! louder! *louder!*——

"Villains!" I shrieked, "dissemble no more! I admit the deed!——tear up the planks!——here, here!——it is the beating of his hideous heart!"

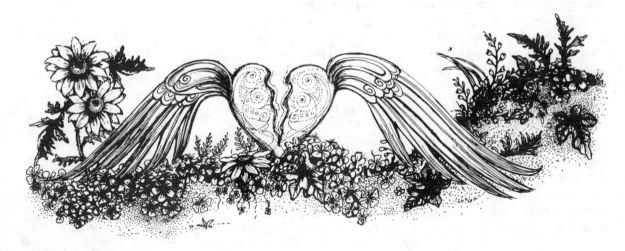

68

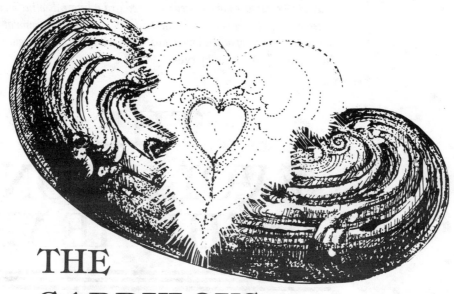

THE GARRULOUS HEART

by Richard Selzer, M.D.

". . . Across the diaphragm and into the chest . . . here at last is all noise; the whisper of the lungs, the *lubdup, lubdup* of the garrulous heart.

"But it is good you do not hear the machinery of your marrow lest it madden like the buzzing of a thousand coppery bees. It is frightening to lie with your ear in the pillow, and hear the beating of your heart. Not that it beats . . . but that it might stop, even as you listen. For anything that moves must come to rest; no rhythm is endless but must one day lurch . . . then halt. Not that it is a disservice to a man to be made mindful of his death, but—at three o'clock in the morning it is less than philosophy. It is Fantasy, replete with dreadful images forming in the smoke of alabaster crematoria. It is then that one thinks of the bristlecone pines, and envies them for having lasted. It is their slowness, I think. Slow down, heart, and drub on."

Aristotle believed that the heart was the source of man's thoughts and emotions, and controlled the rest of the body. This was accomplished through a network of slender threads that linked it to all the other muscles ——and was probably the source of the expression "tugging at one's heart strings."

"Thus nature, ever perfect and divine, doing nothing in vain, has neither given a heart where it was not required, nor produced it before its office had become necessary; but by the same stages in the development of every animal, passing through the forms of all, as I may say (ovum, worm, foetus), it acquires perfection in each."—William Harvey

THE EVOLUTION OF THE HEART

The Sumerians believed the heart to be the site of man's intelligence.

The ancient Hindus believed that by concentrating his meditation upon the heart, the ascetic (or yogi) was able to probe not only his own mind but those of others. The philosopher Shankara says that this concentration should be "in the form of a light the size of the thumb situated in the cavity of the heart."

The first heart was also the simplest. Some 450 million years ago, when life was still restricted to the vast oceans, some tiny primitive creatures had become sufficiently complex to require a circulatory system to pump oxygen throughout their bodies. After a long period of evolution, the first heart developed into a long, narrow vessel that had a regular pulsation. As living things became more complex, the circulatory system kept pace, following a long path that culminated in the most complex, the most efficient, the most spectacularly engineered heart of all, that of mammals.

This development can be retraced by examining the hearts of more ancient forms of life. The ancestral heart could support creatures no more than several inches long. From this first primitive heart and its successors came the two-chambered heart, a heart still found in fish. In the two-chambered heart, blood collects in one chamber and is then propelled into the second chamber, which in turn contracts and pushes the blood out into the circulatory vessels. This heart made it possible for much larger forms of life to develop in the oceans.

The two-chambered heart fulfilled the needs of most sea creatures, but when some species began moving onto the marshy

70

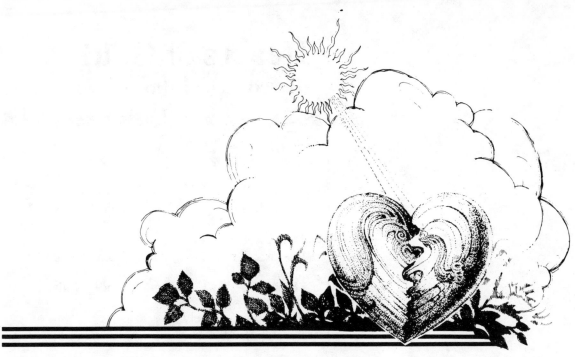

fringes of the land they required a more efficient circulatory system. Creatures of the land developed lungs, which necessitated a rearrangement of the heart. And thus evolved the three-chambered heart still found in amphibians and most reptiles. In this heart, oxygen-rich blood from the lungs is carried to one chamber and oxygen-poor blood coming from the rest of the body enters another. The third chamber draws alternately from each of these two chambers, pumping out oxygen-rich blood to the rest of the body and sending oxygen-poor blood to the lungs to pick up a new supply.

The three-chambered heart emerged about 300 million years ago. Some 100 million years later (give or take 5 million years), the four-chambered heart of the mammals was first developed. Because birds and mammals are warm-blooded, they use up oxygen at a much more rapid rate than other creatures. To meet this pressing need for oxygen, a fourth heart chamber evolved. The existence of this fourth chamber means that oxygen-rich blood and oxygen-poor blood will never mix. Each is sent to a different chamber and routed on its way either to the lungs or the body. This arrangement is much more efficient than the two- or three-chambered heart. It is, in fact, a marvel of engineering that crowns the 300-million-year evolution of the heart.

BEATS PER MINUTE

Blue whale	5-6
Turtle	6-70
Elephant	22-50
Fish	40-80
Human	70-75
Rabbit	100-300
Bird	200-1000
Mouse	300-500
Shrew	500-1000

Hearts of Gold
(Based on a million sales)

Year	Song	Artist
1956	Heartbreak Hotel	Elvis Presley
1957	That's When Your Heartache Begins	Elvis Presley
1963	I Left My Heart in San Francisco	Tony Bennett
1965	Dear Heart	Andy Williams
1967	Sergeant Pepper's Lonely Heart's Club Band	The Beatles
1969	Your Cheatin' Heart	Hank Williams
1969	Put a Little Love in Your Heart	Jackie DeShannon
1969	Happy Heart	Andy Williams
1971	Sweetheart	Englebert Humperdinck
1971	How Can You Mend a Broken Heart?	The Bee Gees
1972	Charley Pride Sings Heart Songs	Charley Pride
1972	Heart of Gold	Neil Young
1973	Heart—It's a Lovebeat	The DeFranco Family
1975	Sheer Heart Attack	Queen
1976	Don't Go Breaking My Heart	Elton John & Kiki Dee
1978	You're Breaking My Heart	Rod Stewart

The Mind lives on the Heart
Like any Parasite—
If that is full of Meat
The Mind is fat.

But if the Heart omit
Emaciate the Wit—
The Aliment of it
So absolute.

—Emily Dickinson

Pickled Venison Heart

1 venison heart
4 quarts water
2 teaspoons salt
1/4 teaspoon poppy seeds
1/4 teaspoon celery seeds
1/4 teaspoon black peppercorns
1 clove garlic, crushed
1 teaspoon thyme
1/2 teaspoon marjoram
1 bay leaf
1 bottle chianti
Horseradish
Jewish pumpernickel

1. Cut a three-quarter-inch slice off the top of the heart. Mix two quarts of the water with one teaspoon of the salt. Soak heart two hours in mixture. Clean out all the blood. Drain.

2. Place heart in a saucepan with remaining water and add the poppy seeds, celery seeds, peppercorns, garlic, thyme, marjoram, bay leaf and remaining salt. Bring to a boil and simmer, covered, until heart is very tender. Cool and let stand in refrigerator two days.

3. Pour off top of broth, leaving about two cups in the bottom with most of the seasonings. Pour in the wine so that it covers the heart and let set in the refrigerator at least a week.

4. Slice very thinly and serve with horseradish and Jewish pumpernickel.
Yield: One dozen to two dozen servings.

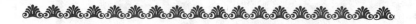

The heart of man is of itself but little, yet great things cannot fill it: it is not big enough at one meal to satisfy a bird, and yet the whole world cannot satisfy it.
—Thomas Dekker

Rabelais, one of the literary masters of old France, was also noted as a doctor. His statements about the heart conform with the prevailing scientific views of his time. In *Pantagruel* he writes: *"The heart doth in its left-side ventricle so thinnify the blood, that it thereby obtains the name of spiritual; which being sent through the arteries to all the members of the body, serveth to warm, and winnow, or fan the other blood which runneth through the veins. The lights never cease with its lappets and bellows to cool and refresh it; in acknowledgment of which good the heart, through the arterial vein, imparts unto it the choicest of its blood. At last it is made so fine and subtle within the rete mirabile, that thereafter those animal spirits are framed and composed of it; by means whereof the imagination, discourse, judgment, resolution, deliberation, ratiocination and memory have their rise, actings, and operations."*

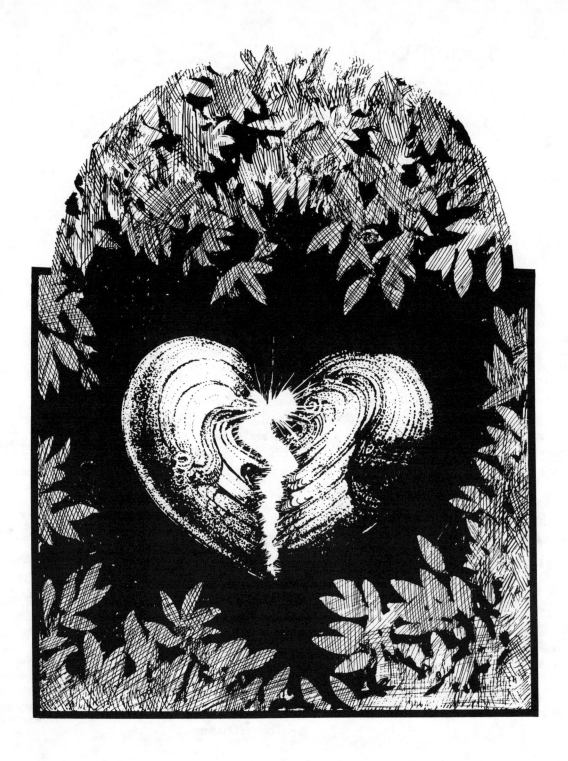

THE BROKEN HEART
by John Donne

He is stark mad, who ever says
   That he hath been in love an hour,
Yet not that love so soon decays,
   But that it can ten in less space devour;
Who will believe me, if I swear
That I have had the plague a year?
   Who would not laugh at me, if I should say
   I saw a flask of powder burn a day?

Ah, what a trifle is a heart,
   If once into love's hands it come!
All other griefs allow a part
   To other griefs, and ask themselves but some;
They come to us, but us Love draws,
He swallows us, and never chaws:
   By him, as by chained shot, whole ranks do die;
   He is the tyrant pike, our hearts the fry.

If 'twere not so, what did become
   Of my heart, when I first saw thee?
I brought a heart into the room,
   But from the room I carried none with me;
If it had gone to thee, I know
Mine would have taught thine heart to show
   More pity unto me: but Love, alas,
   At one first blow did shiver it as glass.

Yet nothing can to nothing fall,
   Nor any place be empty quite,
Therefore I think my breast hath all
   Those pieces still, though they be not unite;
And now, as broken glasses show
A hundred lesser faces, so
   My rags of heart can like, wish, and adore,
   But after one such love, can love no more.

FOR WHAT HIS HEART THINKS HIS TONGUE SPEAKS

William Shakespeare

I here do give thee that, with all my heart
Which, but thou hast already, with all my heart
I would keep from thee.   OTHELLO

. . . Give me that man
That is not passion's slave, and I will wear him
In my heart's core, ay, in my heart of heart,
As I do thee.   HAMLET

He hath a heart as sound as a bell, and his tongue is the clapper; for what his heart thinks his tongue speaks.

MUCH ADO ABOUT NOTHING

What infinite heart's ease
Must kings neglect that private men enjoy!   HENRY V

My heart is turn'd to stone; I strike it, and it hurts my hand.

OTHELLO

My crown is in my heart, not on my head.   3 HENRY VI

What stronger breastplate than a heart untainted!   2 HENRY VI

These words are razors to my wounded heart.   TITUS
ANDRONICUS

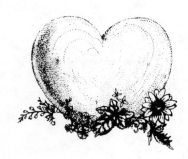

Ferdinand: Here's my hand.
Miranda: And mine, with my heart in't.   THE TEMPEST

Words, words, mere words, no matter from the heart.

TROILUS AND CRESSIDA

Better a little chiding than a great deal of heartbreak.

THE MERRY WIVES OF WINDSOR

. . . 'tis bitter cold
And I am sick at heart.   HAMLET

False face must hide what the false heart doth know.   *MACBETH*

. . . 'Tis not long after
But I will wear my heart upon my sleeve
For daws to peck at.   *OTHELLO*

All offences, my lord, come from the heart; never came any from
mine that might offend your majesty.   *HENRY V*

O tiger's heart wrapp'd in a woman's hide!   *3 HENRY VI*

A goodly apple rotten at the heart.   *MERCHANT OF VENICE*

Now cracks a noble heart. Good night, sweet prince.   *HAMLET*

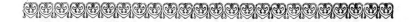

TOWN OF HEART'S CONTENT

HEART'S CONTENT, NEWFOUNDLAND

The original settlers of Newfoundland's Trinity Bay must have been a satisfied lot. On the eastern shore lie the towns of Heart's Desire, Heart's Delight, and Heart's Content. Across the bay, at the mouth of Random Sound, is the village of Little Heart's Ease.

Of the four, only Heart's Content has achieved much notice in the outside world. There, on July 27, 1866, the first transatlantic cable was landed. F.N. Gisborne's original plan had been merely to link St. John's, Newfoundland, with Canada and the United States, but his backer, financier Cyrus Field, had bigger plans. After fifteen years and millions of dollars, they succeeded in linking North America with Europe. And so a small, remote fishing village helped usher in a new era in international communication.

Heart's Content has preserved the original cable station as a museum, and many summer tourists visit the area because of its historic background. Mrs. Alice Cumby, the town clerk, believes there's another reason for Heart's Content's popularity: "According to the older folk of the community, it got its name because the harbor is in the shape of a heart. I guess they added content because you could not come into our beautiful little town without feeling content to stay here."

The heart seine is a weir with a heart-shaped enclosure or pound which can be used to catch fish however the tide may run. The enclosure itself is called a heart net.

In Alberta, Canada, one can find both the Heart River and Heart Lake. On the banks of the latter is the Heart Lake Indian Reserve. Another Heart Lake is located in Ontario, and its shape is astonishingly faithful to its name.

My heart's in the Highlands, my heart is not here,
My heart's in the Highlands, a-chasing the deer;
A-chasing the wild deer, and following the roe,
My heart's in the Highlands wherever I go.

Robert Burns

The HEARTS of AMERICA

Boldt Castle attracts tourists to tiny Heart Island in Jefferson County, New York. One of the Thousand Islands, Heart Island is only two tenths of a mile long; it lies in the St. Lawrence just northwest of Alexandria Bay.

Warwickshire is often called the Heart of England, a name which is derived from its central location in that country.

In America, both the greatest and the smallest heart seem to lie west of the Mississippi. Here the Heart River flows from central North Dakota all the way to the Missouri River at Mandan. Meanwhile, near the Platte River, lies the tiny town of Heartwell in Kearney County, Nebraska.

America's towns and cities have some pretty colorful mottoes, and the heart is one of their favorite symbols. The slogans range all the way from the short and sweet (Brady, Texas, is the Heart of Texas) to the very particular (Augusta, Georgia, the Heart of Eastern Georgia and Western South Carolina); from the poetic (Coeur d' Alene, Idaho, is the Heart of the Emerald Empire in the North Idaho Scenic Land) to the prosaic (Pearson, Georgia, the Heart of the Turpentine Industry); from the historic (Cooperstown, New York, Heart of the Leatherstocking Land) to the practical (Wilkes-Barre, Pennsylvania, Heart of the Valley that Warms a Nation); from the predictable (Heart of the Corn Country, Monona, Iowa) to the unexpected (Heart of the American Riviera, Foley, Alabama).

And of course there are always little disagreements about just who's who. Frankfort, Kentucky; Kansas City, Missouri; and Washington, D.C., all claim to be the Heart of America. But Wahoo, Nebraska and Effingham, Illinois, call themselves the Heart of the Nation and the Heart of the U.S.A. In Florida, Deerfield Beach, Hollywood, and Pompano Beach all lay claim to the title Heart of the Gold Coast. Meanwhile, Somerville and Southbridge, Massachusetts, do battle over the honors for Heart of New England. But lucky Rogers, Arkansas, has no competition for the title Heartland of the Beaver Lake Area.

78

SHAKESPEARE'S SONNETS

The word heart is used 56 times in the 154 poems which make up Shakespeare's famous sonnet sequence. Of these uses, eight occur in a single poem, Sonnet 46, where Shakespeare weaves an elaborate metaphor of litigation in which the heart and the eye contend with one another for rights to the portrait of the young man (Herbert, Earl of Pembroke) who is the subject of the poem:

Mine eye and heart are at a mortal war,
How to divide the conquest of thy sight;
Mine eye my heart thy picture's sight would bar,
My heart mine eye the freedom of that right.
My heart doth plead that thou in him dost lie,
A closet never pierced with crystal eyes,
But the defendant [i.e., eye] doth that plea deny,
And says in him thy fair appearance lies.
To 'cide [decide] this title is impaneled
A quest [jury] of thoughts, all tenants to the heart;
And by their verdict is determined
The clear eye's moiety and the dear heart's part.
  As thus; mine eye's due is thy outward part,
  And my heart's right thy inward love of heart.

Of its fifty-six appearances throughout the sonnets, the word heart appears in a rhyming position—that is, at the end of a line—only seventeen times. On these seventeen euphonious occasions, the word heart is made to rhyme with only three other words: *part* (10 times), *art* (6 times), *depart* (1 time). And speaking of rhymes, one contemporary poet's handbook lists twenty-one modern English words that rhyme with heart. Can you think of more than Shakespeare did?

"It is wisdom to believe the heart."
—George Santayana

"Through our great good fortune, in our youth our hearts were touched with fire."
—Oliver Wendell Holmes, Jr.

HEART'S MAGIC

Sir James Frazer's *The Golden Bough* records many instances of primitive belief in the homeopathic magic of a fleshy diet— better known as a hearty meal.

"In Morocco lethargic patients are given ants to swallow, and to eat lion's flesh will make a coward brave; but people abstain from eating the hearts of fowls, lest thereby they should be rendered timid."

"A North American Indian thought that brandy must be a decoction of hearts and tongues, 'because,' said he, 'after drinking it I fear nothing, and I talk wonderfully.'"

"The Bushmen will not give their children a jackal's heart to eat, lest it should make them timid like the jackal; but they give them a leopard's heart to eat to make them brave like the leopard. When a Wagogo man of East Africa kills a lion, he eats the heart in order to become brave like a lion; but he thinks that to eat the heart of a hen would make him timid."

"The Ainu believe that the heart of the water-ousel is exceedingly wise, and that in speech the bird is most eloquent. Therefore whenever he is killed, he should be at once torn open and his heart wrenched out and swallowed before it has time to grow cold or suffer damage of any kind. If a man swallows it thus, he will become very fluent and wise, and will be able to argue down all his adversaries."

"In Norse legend, Ingiald, son of King Aunund, was timid in his youth, but after eating the heart of a wolf he became very bold; Hialto gained strength and courage by eating the heart of a bear and drinking its blood."

"The Indians of Guayaquil, in Ecuador, used to sacrifice human blood and the hearts of men when they sowed their fields."

Many ancient cultures considered the heart to be the seat of power that controlled other areas of the body. It was believed to be equidistant from the brain and the genitals, and this position enabled it to balance both.

It was considered a great honor among the Iroquois for a warrior to be awarded the heart of a brave prisoner taken in battle. By eating the heart, the victor believed that he would assume some of his enemy's courage.

THE HEART AS SYMBOL

It would be easier to list the cultures in which the heart has *not* been used in a variety of symbolic ways than to enumerate those in which it has attained importance. Throughout recorded history, stylized portraits of the heart have been used in art and literature as symbols of certain qualities and beliefs. Cultures widely distant in both time and place seem to have attributed very similar meanings to the heart.

Again and again, the heart is used to represent the focus, the *center* of a human being, the source from which all intelligence and emotions flow. This perception may have been at least partly based on the early realization of the heart's importance in the body—even the oldest civilizations seem to have known far more about the functionings of the heart than those of the brain. So, just as the physical heart maintained the body, it was thought that the spiritual heart was the source of man's other qualities.

In culture after culture, the heart was given great symbolic importance. And what began as essentially religious beliefs were gradually diffused and adapted in each different culture. In many societies, one or another aspect of the heart became dominant. In the West, the heart became an emblem of lovers, identified as the source of either amorous or religious love. In the East, many cultures came to identify the heart as a symbol of wisdom and spiritual realization.

Progress and change have eroded or entirely eliminated many of these beliefs, but the remnants of such convictions linger on, even if they are only the stereotyped hearts that appear everywhere on that day now set aside for lovers. We still talk easily (though few people would claim to mean it literally) of "broken hearts" and heartsick lovers. Though we may no longer share so many beliefs about the heart, if you were to ask a sampling of people to describe what the heart symbolized, they'd probably tell you some of the same things their ancestors would have.

~~~~~~~~~~~~~~~~~~~~~~~~~~~~~~~~~~~~

The heart has its reasons which reason knows nothing of....We know the truth, not only by the reason, but by the heart.　　　　　—Blaise Pascal

Cave Heart

Veterinary anatomy might be a relatively new field of study, but the cave art of our Paleolithic ancestors some 20,000 years ago shows that the position—and the significance—of the hearts of hunted beasts were well understood. Drawn more or less like the now traditional, symmetrical form with which all disciples of St. Valentine are accustomed, the hearts of the elephant and of the bison, for example, are clearly depicted and accurately placed within the outline drawing of the entire animal form. In these mostly detail-free pictures, the inclusion of the heart bespeaks the caveman's ritualistic belief that the power to conquer an adversary begins to take shape with the ability to capture its image.

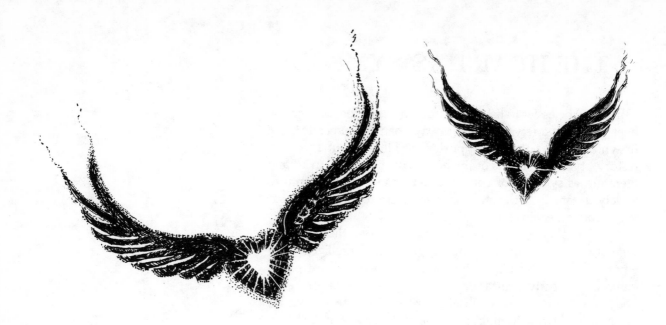

ENTER GIOVANNI
With A Heart Upon His Dagger

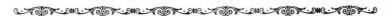

The heart, both as concept and stage prop, is put to frequent use in many of the sensationalistic Renaissance plays. The Elizabethan dramatist John Ford, author of *The Broken Heart* and other grim and powerful plays, identified the heart with all the pleasurable and painful aspects of romantic love. It is mentioned repeatedly in many of his plays, but nowhere is it used more shockingly than in the tragedy *Tis Pity She's a Whore*. The play, first printed in 1633, was one of the most audacious of its time since it concerned the incestuous love between a brother and sister.

Annabella and Giovanni are of a noble family. Both are willful and passionate, and Giovanni gives signs throughout of a morbid, violent temperament. When Annabella becomes pregnant, and he learns that their affair has been discovered, Giovanni murders Annabella. In the excerpt from the climax of the play printed below, Giovanni enters, carrying his sister's (and lover's) heart upon his dagger. The shock of the revelations kills their father, Florio, and Giovanni dies after striking down Annabella's corrupt husband, Sorranzo.

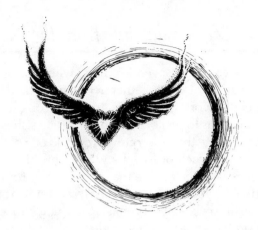

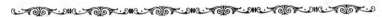

Enter Giovanni with a heart upon his dagger

 GIOVANNI. Here, here, Sorranzo! trimmed in reeking blood,
That triumphs over death, proud in the spoil
Of love and vengeance! Fate, or all the powers
That guide the motions of immortal souls,
Could not prevent me.

 CARDINAL. What means this?

 FLORIO. Son Giovanni!

 GIOVANNI. Be not amazed: if your misgiving hearts
Shrink at an idle sight, what bloodless fear
Of coward passion would have seized your senses,
Had you beheld the rape of life and beauty
Which I have acted!

        . . . 'tis a heart,
A heart my lords, in which is mine entombed:
Tis Annabella's heart . . .

     Have you all no faith
To credit yet my triumphs?
Here I swear
By all that you call sacred, by the love
I bore my Annabella whilst she lived,
These hands have from her bosom ripped this heart.

 CARDINAL. Monster of children! see what thou hast done,
Broke thy old father's heart.

83

The Man Without a Heart

There were once seven brothers, who had neither father nor mother. They lived together in one house and had to do all the household work themselves, to wash, cook, sweep, and whatever else was to be done; for they had no sisters. Of this kind of housekeeping they soon grew tired, and one of them said: "Let us set out, and each of us get a wife." This idea pleased the other brothers, and they made themselves ready for travelling, all excepting the youngest, who preferred to remain at home and keep house, his six brothers promising to bring him a wife with them. The brothers then set out, and all six went forth merrily in the wide world. They soon came into a large, wild forest, where, after wandering about for some time, they found a small house, at the door of which an old man was standing. On seeing the brothers passing by and appearing so gay, he called to them: "For what place are you bound that you pass my door so merrily?" "We are going each of us to fetch a handsome young bride," answered they, "and therefore are we so merry. We are all brothers, but have left one at home, for whom we are also to bring a bride." "I wish you then success in your undertaking," replied the old man; "you see, however, very plainly that I am so lonely that I too have need of a wife, and so I advise you to bring me one also with you." To this the brothers made no answer, but continued on their way, thinking the old man spoke only in jest, and that he could have no occasion for a wife.

They soon arrived in a city, where they found seven young and handsome sisters, of whom each of the brothers chose one, and took the seventh with them for their youngest brother.

When they again arrived in the forest, there stood the old man at his door, apparently awaiting their coming. He even called to them at a distance: "Well, have you brought me a wife with you as I desired you?" "No," answered they, "we could not find one for thee, old man; we have only brought brides for ourselves, and one for our youngest brother." "You must leave her for me," said the old man, "for you must keep to your promise." This the brothers refused to do. The old man then took a little white staff from a shelf over the door, with which when he had touched the six brothers and their brides, they were all turned into gray stones. These, together with the staff, he laid on the shelf above the door, but kept the seventh young bride for himself.

The young woman had now to attend to all that was to be done in the house; and she did it all cheerfully, for what would resistance have availed her? She had, moreover, every comfort with him, the only thought that gave her uneasiness being that he might soon die; for what was she then to do alone in the great wild forest, and how was she to release her six poor enchanted sisters and their betrothed husbands? The longer she lived with him the more dreadful did this thought become; she wept and wailed the whole livelong day, and was incessantly crying in the old man's ear: "Thou art old, and mayest die suddenly, and what am I then to do? I shall be left alone here in this great forest." The old man would then appear sad, and at length said: "Thou hast no cause to be uneasy; I cannot die, for I have no heart in my breast; but even if I should die, the twelve gray stones lie over the house-door, and with them a little white staff. If thou strikest the stones with that staff, thy sisters and their betrothed will again be living." The young woman now appeared contented, and asked him, that as his heart was not in his breast, where he kept it. "My child," answered the old man, "be not so inquisitive; thou canst not know everything." But she never ceased her importunities, until he at last said somewhat peevishly, "Well, in order to make you easy, I tell thee that my heart lies in the coverlet."

Now it was the old man's custom to go every morning into the forest and not return till the evening, when his young house-keeper had to prepare supper for him. One evening on his return, finding his coverlet adorned with all kinds of beautiful feathers and flowers, he asked the young woman the meaning of it. "Oh, father," answered she, "I sit here the whole day alone and can do nothing for thy gratification, and so thought I would do something for the delight of thy heart, which, as thou sayest, is in the coverlet!" "My child," said the old man, laughing, "that was only a joke of mine; my heart is not in the coverlet, it is in a very different place." She then began again to weep and lament, and said: "Thou hast then a heart in thy breast and canst die; what am I then to do, and how shall I recover my friends when thou art dead?" "I tell thee," answered the old man, "that I cannot die, and have positively no heart in my breast; but even if I should die, which is not possible, there lie the gray stones over the door together with

The Man
Without a Heart

a little white stick, with which thou hast only, as I have already told thee, to strike the stones, and thou wilt have all thy friends again!" She then prayed and implored him so long to inform her where he kept his heart, that he at length said: "It is in the room-door."

On the following day she decorated the room-door with variegated feathers and flowers from top to bottom, and when the old man came home in the evening and inquired the cause, she answered: "Oh, father, I sit here the whole day, and can do nothing for thy pleasure, and wished therefore to give some delight to thy heart." But the old man answered as before: "My heart is not in the room-door; it is in a very different place." Then, as on the previous day, she began to weep and implore, and said: "Thou hast then a heart and canst die; thou wilt only deceive me." The old man answered: "Die I cannot; but as thou wilt positively know where my heart is, I will tell thee, that thou mayest be at ease. Far, very far, from here, in a wholly unknown solitary place, there is a large church; this church is well secured by thick iron doors; around it there runs a wide, deep moat; within the church there flies a bird, and in that bird is my heart. So long as that bird lives, I also live. Of itself it will not die, and no one can catch it. Hence I cannot die, and thou mayest be without apprehension."

In the meantime the youngest brother had waited and waited at home; but as his brothers did not return, he supposed that some mishap had befallen them, and therefore set out in quest of them. After traveling for some days he arrived at the house of the old man. He was not at home, but the young woman, his bride, received him. He related to her how he had six brothers, who had all left home to get themselves wives, but that some mischance must have befallen them, as they had never returned. He had, therefore, set out in search of them. The young woman then instantly knew him for her bridegroom, and informed him who she was, and what had become of his brothers and their brides. Both were overjoyed at having thus met; she gave him [food] to eat, and when he had recruited his strength he said: "Tell me now, my dear bride, how I can release my brothers." She then related to him all about the old man, whose heart was not in his breast, but in a far distant church, of which she gave him every particular, according to the old man's narrative. "I will at all events try," said the young man, "whether I cannot get hold of the bird. It is true that the way is long and unknown to me, and the church is well secured; but by God's help I may succeed." "Do so," said the young woman, "seek the bird; for as long as that lives thy brothers cannot be released. This night thou must hide thyself under the bedstead, that the old man may not find thee: tomorrow thou canst continue thy journey." Accordingly he crept under the bed just before the old man's return, and on the following morning, as soon as the old man was gone out, the young woman drew her bridegroom forth from his hiding-place, gave him a whole basketful of provisions, and after a tender farewell, he resumed his journey. He had proceeded a considerable way, when feeling hungry he sat down, placed his basket before him and opened it. While in the act of taking forth some bread and meat, he said: "Let come now every one that desires to eat with me!" At the instant there came a huge red ox, and said: "If thou didst say that every one should come that desires to eat with thee, I would gladly eat with thee." "Very well," said the young man, "I did say so, and thou shalt partake with me." They then began to eat, and when they were satisfied, the red ox, when about to depart, said: "If at any time thou art in difficulty and requirest my aid, thou hast only to utter the wish, and I will come and help thee." He then disappeared among the trees, and the young man recommenced his journey.

When he had proceeded a considerable way farther, he was again hungry, so he sat down, opened his basket, and said as before: "Let those come that desire to eat with me!" In a moment there came from the thicket a large wild boar and said: "Thou hast said that whoever desired to eat with thee should come; now I would gladly eat with thee." The bridegroom answered: "Thou art quite right, comrade; so just fall to." When they had eaten, the boar said: "If thou art ever in difficulty and needest my aid, thou hast only to utter the wish, and I will help thee." He then disappeared in the forest, and the young man pursued his journey.

On the third day, when about to eat, he said again: "Let all that desire to eat with me come!" At the instant a rattling was heard among the trees and a large griffon descended and placed himself by the side of the traveller, saying: "If thou didst say that all who desired to eat with thee might come, I would gladly eat with thee." "With all my heart," answered the bridegroom; "'tis far

The Man
Without a Heart

more pleasant to eat in company than alone; so just fall to." Both then began to eat. When their hunger was satisfied, the griffon said: "If ever thou art in difficulty, thou hast only to call me and I will aid thee." He then disappeared in the air, and the young man went his way.

After travelling a while longer he perceived the church at a distance; so redoubling his pace, he was soon close by it. But now there was the moat in his way, which was too deep for him to wade through and he could not swim. Now the red ox occurred to his recollection: "He could help thee," thought he, "if he were to drink a green path through the water. Oh, that he were here!" Hardly had he expressed the wish when the red ox was there, laid himself on his knees and drank until there was a dry green path through the water. The young man now passed through the moat and stood before the church, the iron doors of which were so strong that he could not force one open, and the walls many feet thick, without an opening in any part. Knowing no other means, he endeavoured to break some stones, one by one out of the wall, and after great labour succeeded in extracting a few. It then occurred to him that the wild boar could help him, and he cried: "Oh, if the wild boar were here!" In an instant it came rushing up, and ran with such force against the wall, that in one moment a large hole was broken through it, and the young man entered the church. Here he saw the bird flying about. "Thou canst not catch it thyself," thought he, "but if the griffon were here——!" Scarcely had he uttered the thought, when the griffon was there; but it cost even the griffon a great deal of trouble to catch the little bird; at last, however, he seized it, gave it into the young man's hand and flew away. Overjoyed, he placed his prize in the basket, and set forth on his way back to the house in which his bride was.

When he reached the house and informed her that he had the bird in his basket, she was overjoyed, and said: "Now thou shalt first eat something in haste, and then creep again under the bed with the bird, so that the old man may know nothing of the matter." This was done, and just as he had crept under the bed, the old man returned home, but felt ill and complained. The young woman then again began to weep, and said: "Ah, now father will die, that I can well see, and he has a heart in his breast!" "Ah, my child," answered the old man, "be still only; I cannot die; it will soon pass over." The bridegroom under the bed now gave the bird a little pinch, and the old man felt quite ill and sat down, and when the young man squeezed it yet harder, he fell to the earth in a swoon. The bride then cried out: "Squeeze it quite to death." The young man did so, and the old man lay dead on the ground. The young woman then drew her bridegroom from under the bed, and afterwards went and took the stones and the little white staff from the shelf over the door, struck every stone with the staff, and in one instant there stood all her sisters and the brothers before her. "Now," said she, "we will set out for home, and celebrate our marriage and be happy; for the old man is dead, and there is nothing more to fear from him." They did so, and lived many years in harmony and happily together.

Pickled Elk's Heart

1   elk's heart, well cleaned
2   teaspoons whole cloves
1   bay leaf
4   cups cider vinegar
1   tablespoon salt
1   onion, sliced
1/2 teaspoon dry mustard

1. Place the elk's heart in a deep saucepan and cover with water. Bring to a boil, cover and simmer until tender, about three hours.

2. Measure two cups of the cooking liquid and add remaining ingredients to it. Bring to a boil and cool.

3. Drain the heart and place in the cooled vinegar mixture so that heart is submerged. Soak ten days to two weeks in a cool place. Slice thinly.

4. *Yield:* One dozen servings.

The Happiest Heart

"The happiest heart that ever beat
  Was in some quiet breast
That found the common daylight sweet,
  And left to Heaven the rest."

—John V. Cheney

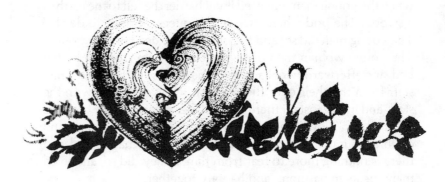

YOU WILL MEET A TALL, WARM-HEARTED STRANGER

"There is no instinct like that of the heart."
—Lord Byron

"There is only one quality worse than hardness of heart and that is softness of head."
—Theodore Roosevelt

"The wrinkles of the heart are more incredible than those of the brow."—Deluzy

"A kind heart is a fountain of gladness, making everything in its vicinity to freshen into smiles."
—Washington Irving

Tarot decks are the ancestors of today's playing cards, so it's not surprising that a belief in special powers should still be attached to our modern hearts, spades, clubs, and diamonds. Although many different tarot cards are available, some psychics prefer to use a regular deck of playing cards when they attempt to read the future.

The cards are shuffled and then arranged in a pattern similar to that used in a traditional Tarot reading. Although it's been said that the cards only focus the seer's energies and don't in themselves carry a message, various systems of meanings have been worked out so that anyone can use a deck of cards to "read" the future.

Cards say different things depending on how they come out of a deal. A king, for instance, has one meaning if it's right side up, another if it comes out of the deck upside down, or reversed. There are also several systems for determining these meanings, and their interpretations are sometimes quite at variance.

Bearing all this in mind, here are some messages your hearts might be sending you.

ACE   Untroubled family life.
       Reversed: Quarrelsome, difficult family life.

KING   A fair-haired, easy-going man will have an influence
       in your future.
       Reversed: In your future there is an exacting individual
       who is difficult to get along with.

QUEEN A fair-haired woman, virtuous and true, will have
       some part in your life.
       Reversed: Trouble lies ahead in the path of love.

JACK   A loyal, kindly young man will be involved in your
       life.
       Reversed: Loyal, kind-hearted thoughts directed at
       you, or directed outward by you.

TEN   A symbol of one's work and/or of love.
       Reversed: An unexpected and pleasant event is likely.

NINE   Success. A harmonious life. Contentment.
       Reversed: Obstacles or worries will block your path.

EIGHT An unexpected visit is likely—or a present.
       Reversed: An auburn-haired young woman will be
       connected in some pleasant way with your future.

SEVEN The thoughts of a loved one are with you.
       Reversed: The hopes and desires of a loved one will in-
       fluence your course of action.

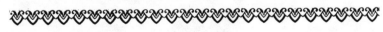 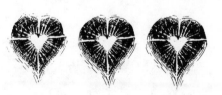

LIMERICK

There was a sad merchant of tarts
Whose horses came after his carts;
*   When asked about this*
*   He replied, with a kiss,*
That heart-strings are known to push hearts.

The Honorable Heart of La Tour d'Auvergne

Among the proverbial landmarks in the life and death of the eighteenth-century French soldier La Tour d'Auvergne (b. 1743), the disposition of his courageous heart is not likely to be forgotten. Napoleon Bonaparte led the entire French army in a three-day period of mourning after the heroic death of this "First Grenadier of France" in the year 1800. La Tour's surviving comrades in the military took up a collection to purchase a silver urn in which the hero's heart was placed. The prized vessel was for many years borne by the company of the 46th Grenadiers, who eventually entrusted it to Garibaldi. Eventually, in 1883, the noble heart was placed in the custody of the city of Paris.

First in the Hearts

It was the *Resolutions Presented to the House of Representatives* upon the death of George Washington that carried Henry Lee's famous dedication, "To the memory of the Man, first in war, first in peace, and first in the hearts of his countrymen."

A HEARTBEAT AWAY

"U.S. history to date has shown that there are better than two chances in ten that the president's heartbeat will stop during his term of office."—William Safire

U.S. presidents whose hearts stopped beating in office:

> William H. Harrison
> Zachary Taylor
> Abraham Lincoln
> James A. Garfield
> William McKinley
> Warren G. Harding
> Franklin D. Roosevelt
> John F. Kennedy

"The Republican Vice Presidential candidate . . . asks you to place him a heartbeat away from the Presidency."—Adlai Stevenson

Heart Attack Market

Peter Wyckoff's Dictionary of Stock Market Terms (Prentice-Hall, 1968) defines "heart attack market" as "the sharp sell-off on Monday, September 26, 1955, caused by President Eisenhower's heart attack. The Dow-Jones Industrial Average dropped 6.5%, or 31.89 points on a volume of 7.7 million shares, their greatest one-day decline since October 28, 1929."

HEARTBROKEN

Some leisurely paging through *Stedman's Medical Dictionary* will yield the following assortment of hearts:

Armored heart: calcareous deposits in the pericardium occurring in subacute or chronic inflammation.

Beer-heart: a hypertrophied heart supposedly due to the greater "load" resulting from an excessive consumption of fluids.

Bony heart: the presence of more or less extensive calcareous patches in the pericardium and walls of the heart.

Forward heart failure: the theory of forward failure maintains that the phenomena of congestive heart failure result from the inadequate cardiac output, and especially from the consequent inadequacy of renal blood flow with resulting retention of sodium and water.

Hairy heart: pericarditis in which the heart is seen post mortem to be covered with a shaggy, fibrinous exudate; cor hirsutum; cor tomentosum; trichocardia; shaggy pericardium.

Heart hurry: rapid action of the heart; tachycardia.

Icing heart: pericarditis in which the heart is seen post mortem covered with a thick, white coat like the icing of cake.

Irritable heart: soldier's heart; neurocirculatory asthenia; a cardiac neurosis marked by rapid pulse, dyspnea, and various anxiety symptoms, associated with an increased susceptibility to fatigue.

Skin heart: the peripheral blood vessels.

Tiger heart: a fatty degenerated heart in which the fat is disposed in the form of broken stripes.

Tobacco heart: cardiac irritability marked by irregular action, palpitation, and sometimes pain, occurring as a result of the excessive use of tobacco.

Waist of the heart: in the chest x-ray, the middle segment of the cardiac silhouette, containing the pulmonary salient.

The heartworm is a parasite which infects dogs.

Heartwater sickness is a disease of south and central Africa occurring in cattle, sheep, and goats.

The longest heart stoppage in a living human being was recorded on January 8, 1977. After 3 hours and 32 minutes, Miss Jean Jawbone, 20, was revived by a team of 17 at the Winnipeg Medical Centre in Manitoba, Canada.

The Heart as a Religious Symbol

Almost every major religion has made use of the heart as a symbol. It's worthwhile to note that accurate physiological information was the basis for this use. Heart failure, fainting caused by heart malfunction, and wounds of the heart, are all described accurately in the books of the Old Testament. In addition, the relation of a healthy heart to longevity, the manner in which the heart functions, and its centrality in the functions of the body, are also mentioned. These descriptions indicate a high level of knowledge about the physical workings of the heart among Near Eastern cultures as long as 2,500 years ago.

In the Old Testament, the heart is understood to be the center and source of each human being, the point from which thought, emotions, and will all emanate, and the organ which focuses the function of conscience. It is from the heart that all a person's actions originate. Understanding, imagination, determination, and memory all have their origin in the heart. Virtue and vice, humility and pride, good and evil thoughts and deeds, all come from the heart.

This belief in the primacy of the heart was carried through into the New Testament, and was adopted as a tenet of the Christian church as it was first formed. Indeed, the heart is referred to repeatedly by Jesus—the "pure in heart" are those who will see God; people having "honest and good" hearts are the soil in which the seeds of righteousness will grow. Hidden within the heart are those qualities which will reveal the person to be either pure or impure. And only God can read the truth engraved in each heart.

The heart is also a familiar motif in religious art. In Christianity it is often a symbol of love, piety, and charity. Abstract renderings of the heart have been adapted as ornaments to church architecture, but the heart's main use is as a symbol in painting and sculpture. A flaming heart is meant to communicate religious fervor, and when held in the hands of a saint, it symbolizes human love of God.

The image of the Sacred Heart of Jesus, represented as a flam-

The Heart Is the Mind's Bible

. . . I will call the world a School instituted for the purpose of teaching little children to read—I will call the human heart the horn Book used in that School—and I will call the Child able to read, the Soul made from that school and its hornbook . . . Not merely is the Heart a Hornbook, It is the Minds Bible, it is the Minds experience, it is the teat from which the Mind or intelligence sucks its identity. —John Keats

ing heart, probably dates back to the early Middle Ages. It has an important place in the sacred art of the Jesuits, in which Jesus is sometimes shown parting his garments to reveal the flaming heart in the middle of his breast. The flaming heart surrounded by thorns is also used to represent the Sacred Heart of Jesus, while the flaming heart pierced by seven knives represents the sorrows of the Blessed Virgin.

When the flaming heart is pierced by an arrow, it symbolizes repentance of sin and devotion to faith under great trials. Both the flaming heart and a heart pierced by an arrow are attributes of St. Augustine. The heart is also associated with St. Theresa and St. Bernadine. When the heart is seen with a cross, it refers to the story in which Christ appeared in a vision to St. Katherine of Siena and replaced her heart with his own.

Religious symbolism has carried over into the secular world. For instance, a heart shown with a cross and anchor usually means that love has been joined with faith and a belief in the future. And a heart pierced by Cupid's arrow is, of course, the familiar sign of romantic love.

"The hearts of holy men are temples in the truth of things, and, in type and shadow, they are heaven itself."—Jeremy Taylor

"But what comes out of the mouth proceeds from the heart, and this defiles a man. For out of the heart come evil thoughts, murder, adultery, fornication, theft, false witness, slander."
—Matthew 15:18

"The heart is deceitful above all things, and desperately wicked."—Jeremiah 17:9

Where Your Treasure Is, There Will Your Heart Be Also

In his *Lives of the Saints* (1623), Edward Kinesman tells how "St. Anthony of Pauda, preaching a funeral sermon over a rich man of very penurious habits, took for his text *Where your treasure is, there will your heart be also*. St. Anthony said, 'This is obviously true, inasmuch as the heart of the deceased would not be found in his dead body, but in his moneybags.' Search being made, sure enough there was no heart in the dead body, but in one of the largest of the moneybags there was the dead man's heart, as fresh as if it had only that moment been removed from the carcass."

Proverbs

Keep thy heart with all diligence; for out of it are the issues of life.

The heart knoweth his own bitterness: and a stranger doth not intermeddle with his joy.

Even in laughter the heart is sorrowful.

He that is of a merry heart hath a continual feast.

A man's heart deviseth his way: but the Lord directeth his steps.

A merry heart doeth good like a medicine.

As he thinketh in his heart, so is he.

He that trusteth in his own heart is a fool.

Give strong drink unto him that is ready to perish, and wine unto those that be of heavy hearts.

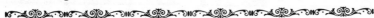

Man looketh at the outward appearance but the Lord looketh on the heart.
—I Samuel 16:17

The heart of a man changeth his countenance, whether it be for good or evil.
—Ecclesiasticus 10:7

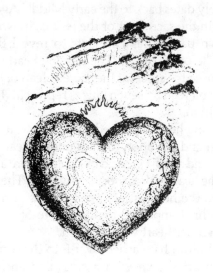

THE HEART OF MIDLOTHIAN

In 1817 the Heart of Midlothian—undoubtedly more familiar to its inmates as the Tolbooth, the city prison of Edinburgh—was razed. A passage from Sir Walter Scott's novel *The Heart of Midlothian* (1818) begins as two men are explaining the dubious nomenclature to a third. Their conversation quickly turns into a contest in verbally out-hearting one another:

> *"Then the Tolbooth of Edinburgh is called the Heart of Midlothian?"*
> *"So termed and reputed, I assure you."*
> *"I think," said I, with the bashful diffidence with which a man lets slip a pun in the presence of his superiors, "the metropolitan county may, in that case, be said to have a sad heart."*
> *"Right as my glove, Mr. Pattieson," added Mr. Hardie; "and a close heart, and a hard heart—keep it up, Jack."*
> *"And a wicked heart, and a poor heart," answered Halkit, doing his best.*
> *"And yet it may be called in some sort a strong heart, and a high heart," rejoined the advocate. "You see I can put you both out of heart."*
> *"I have played all my hearts," said the younger companion.*

During World War II, Parry Island, the Eniwetok Atoll, and the Marshall Islands were referred to by the code name "heartstrings."

96

HEARTY QUOTES QUIZ

Match the poets with the hearty quotes below.

a. Charlotte Bronte
b. Lewis Carroll
c. Emily Dickinson
d. John Keats
e. Andrew Marvell

f. John Donne
g. William Shakespeare
h. Percy Shelley
i. Sir John Suckling
j. William Butler Yeats

(1) *An age at least to every part*
    And the last age should show your heart.

(2) *Batter my heart, three-personed God . . .*

(3) *A pity beyond all telling*
    Is hid in the heart of love.

(4) *My heart aches, and a drowsiness numbness pains*
    My sense, as though of hemlock I had drunk . . ..

(5) *It is not, nor it cannot come to good,*
    But break my heart, for I must hold my tongue.

(6) *The human heart has hidden treasures,*
    In secret kept, in silence sealed.

(7) *One by one, and two by two,*
    He toss'd them human hearts to chew.

(8) *I prithee send me back my heart,*
    *   Since I cannot have thine;*
    For if from yours you will not part,
    *   Why then shouldst thou have mine?*

(9) *The mind lives on the heart*
    Like any parasite.

(10) *And my heart is like nothing so much as a bowl*
     Brimming over with quivering curds.

ANSWERS: (1), e; (2), f; (3), j; (4), d; (5), g; (6), a; (7), h; (8), i; (9), c; (10), b.

"The heart is an astrologer that always divines the truth."—Calderon

"The great conservative is the heart."
    —Nathaniel Hawthorne

"When the heart is on fire, some sparks fly out of the mouth."—Homer

"The heart of a wise man should resemble a mirror, which reflects every object without being sullied by any."—Confucius

97

Unlearn'd, he knew no schoolman's subtle art,
No language, but the language of the heart.

—Alexander Pope

The Language of the Heart

If an international gossip column reported the exchange of *hjerte* for *sziv* between a Danish lady and a Hungarian gentleman, we'd have to suppose that some kind of knot had been tied: perhaps the suturing-up after a bit of fancy surgery—perhaps the intertwining of amorous souls.

Arabic	qalb (*tr*)	*Italian*	cuore
Czech	srdce	*Norwegian*	hjerte
Danish	hjerte	*Polish*	serce
Dutch	hart	*Portuguese*	coracao
Esperanto	koro	*Rumanian*	inima
Finnish	sydan	*Russian*	syertse (*tr*)
French	coeur	*Serbo-Croatian*	srce
German	herz	*Spanish*	corazon
Greek	kardia (*tr*)	*Swahili*	moyo
Hebrew	lev (*tr*)	*Swedish*	hjarta
Hungarian	sziv	*Turkish*	kalb
Indonesian	annutdjg	*Yiddish*	herts (*tr*)

tr—transliteration

Heart-to-Heart

In 1968, Myron Brenton published a book entitled *Sex and Your Heart* in which he cited some very interesting new research. One study, conducted by Boas and Goldschmidt, measured the heart rate of a couple engaged in sex and concluded what many people had already suspected—that intercourse can be one of the most strenuous activities around.

The average resting heart rate is about 70 beats per minute, but when the subjects of the study began their sexual activity their heart rates were already at 90, and these rates reached higher levels with each orgasm, eventually climbing to almost 150. Certainly more taxing than a cold shower, which averages a maximum heart rate of somewhere around 105!

"An advantage of having a hard heart is that it will take a lot to break it."—W. Burton Baldry

"Nothing is less in our power than the heart, and far from commanding we are forced to obey it."
—J.J. Rousseau

"In each human heart are a tiger, a pig, an ass, and a nightingale. Diversity of character is due to their unequal activity."—Ambrose Bierce

98

LOVE, THEFT, and the HEART

". . . She has seen clearly the treachery of him who pretended he was a faithful lover while he was a false and treacherous thief. This thief has traduced my lady, who was ill prepared for any evil, and to whom it never occurred that he would steal her heart away. Those who love truly do not steal hearts away; there are, however, some men, by whom these former are called thieves, who themselves go about deceitfully making love, but in whom there is no real knowledge of the matter. The lover takes his lady's heart, of course, but he does not run away with it; rather does he treasure it against those thieves who, in the guise of honourable men, would steal it from them. But those are deceitful and treacherous thieves who vie with one another in stealing hearts for which they care nothing. The true lover, wherever he may go, holds the heart dear and brings it back again."

—Chretien de Troyes

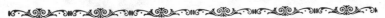

We call the committing of a thing to memory the getting it by heart, for it is the memory that must transmit it to the heart; and it is in vain to expect that the heart should keep its hold of any truth, when the memory has let it go.

—Robert South

OF DREAMS and the HEART

While Sigmund Freud reports that hollow boxes or baskets in certain dreams may represent the heart, *Zolar's Encyclopedia and Dictionary of Dreams* tells us just what to expect from the various appearances of the heart in our dreams. A dream in which you are eating heart meat, Zolar declares, portends a happy love affair; and to dream of cooking heart meat signifies a successful future. Should you dream of losing your heart, it's not a romance—it means that death is near. Dreaming of having a wounded heart relates to marital separation, while dreaming of the heart of an unmarried person suggests elopement and marriage. And those of our readers who are plagued by dreams of being breathless due to heart trouble, should take heart—Zolar says it means you will surpass your friends.

"There is an awful warmth about my heart like a load of immortality."—John Keats

"Look into any man's heart you please, and you will always find, in every one, at least one black spot which he has to keep concealed."

—Henrik Ibsen

"Cruelty has a human heart."—William Blake

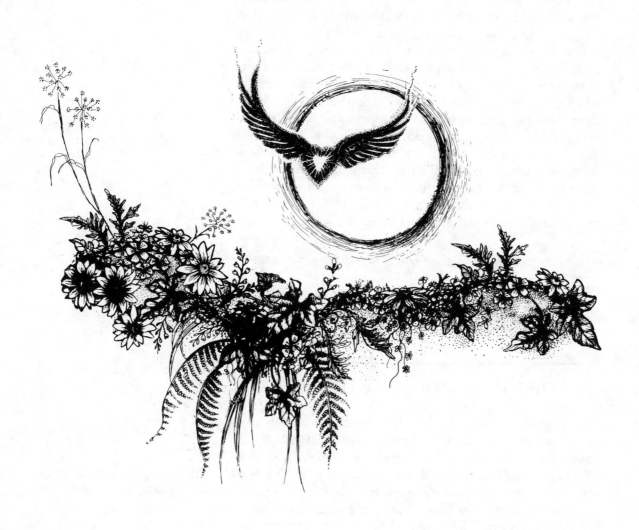

HEARTBREAK HILL

A NEW ENGLAND FOLKTALE
told by Samuel Adams Drake

Turning away from the town through unfrequented bylanes, all green and spotted with daisies, let us ascend Heartbreak Hill in the southeast corner. The view is certainly charming. The reader asks what we see; and, like one on a tower, we reply: In the distance, across a lonely waste of marshes, through which glistening tidal streams crawl on their bellies among reeds, and sun their glossy backs among sand-dunes, we see the bald Ipswich Hundreds, a group of smooth, gray-green, desolate-looking hills stretched along the coast. They are isolated by these marshes from the mainland, which they seem trying to rejoin. Through the openings between these hills we catch the glitter of a ragged line of sand-dunes heaped up like snow-drifts at the edge of the shore, over which rises the sea, and the harbor-bar, overspread with foam.

It being a clear day, we can see from Cape Ann as far as Cape Neddock, and all that lies or floats between; but for leagues the coast is sad and drear, and from the sand, intrenching it everywhere with a natural dyke, the eye turns gratefully upon the refreshing sea. Then, as the Maine coast sweeps gracefully round to the east, the blue domes of Agamenticus rise above it, while the long dark land-line shoots off into the ocean, diminishing gradually from the mountain, like a musical phrase whose last note we strive to catch long after it has died away.

Beneath us is a narrow valley through which a river runs with speed. The town occupies both banks, which rise into considerable eminences above it. All around are the evidences of long occupation of the land,—fields that have borne crops, and trees that have been growing for centuries; houses whose steep roofs descend almost to the ground; graveyards whose mossed stones lean this way and that with age. Finally, the traditions that we are unwilling to see expire, cast a pleasing glamour over the place,—

Heartbreak Hill

something like the shadows which the ancient elms fling down upon the hot and dusty roads.

The river shoots through the gray arches of a picturesque stone bridge out upon the broad levels of marsh land stretching seaward. Through these it loiters quietly along down to the sea. At the town it is an eager mill-stream; at the ocean it is as calm as a mill-pond. The tide brings in a few fishing-boats, but seldom anything larger; for it is no longer an avenue of commerce, as in bygone days.

The oldest of Ipswich legends is associated with this hill, and accounts for its name, though the obscurity surrounding its origin baffles any attempt to trace it to an authentic source. The name is however found upon the earliest records of the town, and it is probably as old as the settlement, which was begun by the whites in 1635 as a check to the expected encroachments of Cardinal Richelieu's colony, then established in Acadia. But before this, we know, from Captain Smith, that the place was the most populous Indian settlement in all Massachusetts Bay, it being the seat of a powerful sagamore, and known by its Indian name of Agawam. That a few white people were living among the Indians here previous to 1635 is evident from the tenor of one of the first recorded acts of the new Colony, dated September 7, 1630, commanding those that were planted at Agawam forthwith to come away. It is perhaps to this early time that the legend of Heartbreak Hill refers, since it is known that the Agawams were a docile and hospitable people, who welcomed the coming of the English among them with open arms; and it is also known that the place was more or less frequented by the English fishing-ships.

Briefly, the legend relates the romantic story of an Indian maiden who fell in love with a white sailor, and upon his sailing for a distant land, she used to climb this hill and pass her days sitting upon the summit watching for his return. But the months and years passed without bringing any tidings of him. He never did come back; and still the deserted one watched and waited, until she pined away, and at length died of a broken heart. There is a ledge on the summit where the Indian girl sat watching for her lover's return; and when she died, her lonely grave was made by the side of it. By others the legend is differently related. Some say that as the girl one day wended her way wearily to the top of the hill, she saw her lover's vessel making the desperate attempt to

102

gain the port in the height of a violent gale. But it drove steadily on among the breakers, and was dashed to pieces and swallowed up before her eyes. In her poem Mrs. Thaxter adopts the former version, which, if less tragic, appeals in a more subtle way to our sympathies. In any case the hill has become a monument to faithful affection, and as such is the favorite resort of lovers in all the country round.

HEARTBREAK HILL

by Celia Thaxter

In Ipswich town, not far from the sea,
    Rises a hill which the people call
Heartbreak Hill, and its history
    Is an old, old legend, known to all.

It was a sailor who won the heart
    Of an Indian maiden, lithe and young;
And she saw him over the sea depart,
    While sweet in her ear his promise rung;

For he cried, as he kissed her wet eyes dry,
    "I'll come back, sweetheart; keep your faith!"
She said, "I will watch while the moons go by."
    Her love was stronger than life or death.

So this poor dusk Ariadne kept
    Her watch from the hill-top rugged and steep;
Slowly the empty moments crept
    While she studied the changing face of the deep,

Fastening her eyes upon every speck
    That crossed the ocean within her ken;
Might not her lover be walking the deck,
    Surely and swiftly returning again?

The Isles of Shoals loomed, lonely and dim,
    In the northeast distance far and gray,
And on the horizon's uttermost rim
    The low rock heap of Boone Island lay.

Oh, but the weary, merciless days,
    With the sun above, with the sea afar,—
No change in her fixed and wistful gaze
    From the morning-red to the evening star!

Like a slender statue carved of stone
    She sat, with hardly motion or breath.
She wept no tears and she made no moan,
    But her love was stronger than life or death.

He never came back! Yet, faithful still,
    She watched from the hill-top her life away.
And the townsfolk christened it Heartbreak Hill,
    And it bears the name to this very day.

MOPPING
YOUR HEARTACHES AWAY

A study by Dr. Ralph S. Paffenberger of Stanford University School of Medicine indicates that strenuous exercise will decrease the chances of heart attack. The following activities in increasing value of heart-attack prevention are indicated:

(1) Strolling at 1 m.p.h. and walking at 2 m.p.h.

(2) Golf, using a power cart.

(3) Cleaning windows, mopping floors, and vacuuming.

(4) Bowling.

(5) Walking at 3 m.p.h. and cycling at 6 m.p.h.

(6) Golf, using a pull-cart.

(7) Scrubbing floors.

(8) Walking at 3.5 m.p.h. and cycling at 8 m.p.h.

(9) Golf, carrying clubs.

(10) Tennis doubles.

(11) Walking at 4 m.p.h., cycling at 10 m.p.h., and ice or roller skating.

(12) Walking at 5 m.p.h. and cycling at 11 m.p.h.

(13) Tennis singles.

(14) Jogging at 5 m.p.h. and cycling at 12 m.p.h.

(15) Downhill skiing.

(16) Running at 5.5 m.p.h. and cycling at 13 m.p.h.

(17) Running at 6 or more m.p.h.

(18) Swimming.

During the Korean War, Heartbreak Hill was the scene of heavy fighting in September and October of 1951.

The Indians at Hudson's Bay called the magpie the heart bird because of the shape of the large black area on its breast.

"It is more fatal to neglect the heart than the head."—Theodore Parker

~~~~~~

If you forgive people enough you belong to them, and they to you, whether either person likes it or not—squatter's rights of the heart.

—James Hilton

A MANY-HEARTED GARDEN

The wild ginger, *Asarum canadense*, or Canada snakeroot, is also known as *heart snakeroot*.

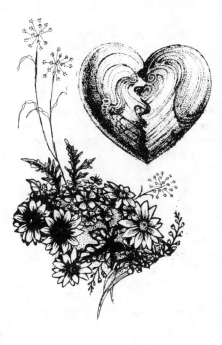

The spotted medic, Medicago maculata, is also known as the *heart trefoil* because of its obcordate leaflets and the somewhat heart-shaped purple or flesh-colored spot on each leaflet. It is also called *heart clover* or *heart leaf.*

The plant self-heal, *Brunella vulgaris*, is also called *heart-of-the-earth.*

Heart pea or *heartseed* is a general name of plants of the genus *Cardio-spermum* (the English name is a translation of the Greek), but more especially of *C. halicacabum*, a beautiful vine well known among horticulturists. In the United States it is called the balloon vine, a name derived from its large, triangular, inflated fruit. The genus takes its name from the white, heart-shaped scar which marks the attachment of the seed.

Heart shake is a defect in timber that occurs when one or more splits cross the center of a tree.

When the wood in a tree begins to die and the walls of its cells harden, it is called *heartwood*. Heartwood is of no use to a tree except as a support. Because of its hardness and dryness, it is frequently used for industrial purposes.

The *heart-leaved tway-blade* is a small orchid found in the British Isles and North America.

The salad known as *heart of palm* is made from the buds of the cabbage palmetto.

The *heartnut, Juglans sieboldiana cordiformis*, is also known as the Japanese walnut.

Sweet cherries are sometimes called *heart cherries* because of their shape.

"Stands the lilac bush tall-growing with heart-shaped leaves of rich green."—Walt Whitman

Heartweed, or Polygonum persicaria, is named for the heart-shaped markings on its leaves.

The heart urchin is a heart-shaped sea urchin. The name describes any spatangoid. The heart urchin is also sometimes know as mermaid's head.

The heart shell is a bivalve mollusk of the family Isocardiidae or Glossidae. The name Isocardia cor comes from the heart-shaped contour of the valves when viewed from the front.

STATISTICS
from the
AMERICAN HEART ASSOCIATION

Of the 24 million Americans suffering from high blood pressure, at least 7 million are not even aware that they have the problem.

One out of every four heart attack deaths occurs to someone under the age of 65; one out of every six stroke victims is under the age of 65.

Heart disease and its widespread effects cost the country about 28 billion dollars a year.

The Warning Signals of a Heart Attack

According to the American Heart Association, the following symptoms are signs of a heart attack:
—Uncomfortable pressure, fullness, or squeezing associated with pain in the center of the chest, lasting two minutes or more.
—Pain spreading to the shoulders, neck, or arms.
—Severe pain, dizziness, fainting, sweating, nausea, or shortness of breath. Sharp, stabbing twinges of pain do not usually accompany a heart attack.

About one million Americans die every year as a result of cardiovascular disease—half of all the deaths in this country. The term cardiovascular disease (CVD) refers to ailments that afflict the heart, including heart attacks, strokes, hypertension, and heart defects. Here is the fatality breakdown for 1976:

646,073	died of heart attacks
188,623	died of strokes
16,820	died of hypertensive disease
13,110	died of rheumatic heart disease
6,279	died of congenital heart defects

More than 29,000,000 Americans suffer from some form of heart disease. Of that number:

24,000,000	suffer from hypertension
4,120,000	have coronary heart disease
1,840,000	suffer from the after-effects of strokes
1,800,000	have rheumatic heart disease

The danger of a heart attack or stroke increases with the number of risk factors present. Among these factors are the heavy, regular use of cigarettes; a diet that includes large amounts of cholesterol; and hypertension. For instance, a man smoking more than a pack of cigarettes a day runs twice the risk of a heart attack and five times the risk of a stroke of a nonsmoker. A man having a blood pressure reading over 150 has twice the likelihood of a heart attack and four times the risk of a stroke of a man whose blood pressure is under 120. And a man with a blood cholesterol level of 250 or more has three times the risk of a heart attack and stroke of a man with a cholesterol level below 194.

Art is long, and Time is fleeting,
* And our hearts, though stout and brave,*
Still, like muffled drums, are beating
* Funeral marches to the grave.*
—Henry Wadsworth Longfellow

If we had a keen vision of all that is ordinary in human life, it would be like hearing the grass grow or the squirrel's heart beat, and we should die of that roar which is the other side of silence.

—George Eliot

Sounds the Heart Makes

Few sounds are as familiar to us as that of the heartbeat. It is one of the first (perhaps *the* first) sound we hear, and throughout life it remains readily identifiable. But what exactly is it? The "lubb dubb" sound of the heart comes from vibrations passing outward from the heart into the chest wall. The first heart sound ("lubb") is produced by the backflow of blood in the ventricles when the ventricular valves close. As the valves close, blood that has been surging forward is suddenly driven back. This sets up a vibration in the walls of the ventricles, and the vibration travels outward, passing into the chest wall where it is attached to the heart. The vibration in the chest wall creates sound waves which, when monitored with the aid of a stethoscope, sound very much like "lubb."

The second heart sound ("dubb") is created by the vibrations caused by the forceful reverberation of the blood between the arterial walls and the heart valves when the pulmonic and aortic semilunar valves shut. These vibrations, different in tenor from the vibrations set up in the ventricles, pass into the chest wall, are transformed into sound waves, and come out sounding like "dubb."

The "dubb" follows "lubb" after only a brief pause. But a pause twice as long occurs between "dubb" and the next "lubb." During the pause the valves are open, and the blood that passes through them is silent to our ears.

...when your heart begins to bleed,
You're dead, and dead, and dead, indeed.
—Early English Nursery Rhyme

107

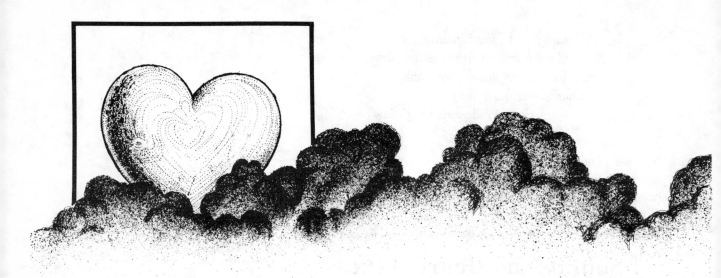

Words, Words, Mere Words,
No Matter from the Heart

They are not dead who live
In hearts they leave behind.—Hugh Robert Orr

Faint heart never won fair lady.—William S. Gilbert

Absence makes the heart grow fonder.—Thomas Haynes Bayly

Bury my heart at wounded knee.—Stephen Vincent Benet

My heart is a lonely hunter that hunts on a lonely hill.—Fiona Macleod

The same heart beats in every breast.—Matthew Arnold

We should count time by heart-throbs.—Philip James Bailey

The logic of the heart is absurd.—Julie de Lespinasse

A love-sick heart dies when the heart is whole,
For all the heart's health is to be sick with love.—Edward P. Mathers

The dictates of the heart are the voice of fate. —Johan von Schiller

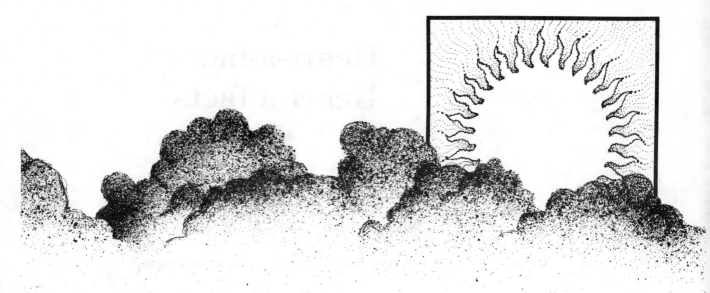

The way to a man's heart is through his stomach.—Fanny Fern

A starved heart deserves at least one crumb during a year.—O. Henry

When the heart speaks, glory itself is an illusion.—Napoleon

The heart of the fool is in his mouth, but the mouth of the wise man is in his heart.—Benjamin Franklin

Absinthe makes the heart grow fonder.—Addison Mizner

The heart has arguments with which the understanding is not acquainted.
—Ralph Waldo Emerson

For where your treasure is, there will your heart be also.—Matthew 6:21

The hardest trial of the heart is, whether it can bear a rival's failure without triumph.—Conrad Aiken

What the heart has once owned and had, it shall never lose.
—H.W. Beecher

A noble heart, like the sun, showeth its greatest countenance in its lowest estate.—Sir Philip Sidney

Memory, wit, fancy, acuteness, cannot grow young again in old age; but the heart can.—J.P. Richter

Heart-a-facts
Heart-a-facts

The smaller the mammal, the faster the heartbeat.

The heart of a shrew beats about 1000 times a minute.

The heart of the largest blue whale weighs about 1000 pounds. This heart beats about 5 or 6 times a minute.

An earthworm has ten hearts.

The mature human heart weighs about 10 to 12 ounces and is about 5 1/2 inches long, 4 inches wide, and 3 inches thick.

The word heart appears 1,284 times in this book.

The heart rate is higher on warmer days.

As a functioning muscle, the heart extracts about 70% of the oxygen carried in the blood to nourish its own beating mechanism.

Courage and cordiality come from heart.

Thirty-five percent of all the fuel for the heart is derived from lactic acid.

The heart rate increases after a heavy meal.

In a minute, a woman's heart beats usually 7 or 8 times more than a man's.

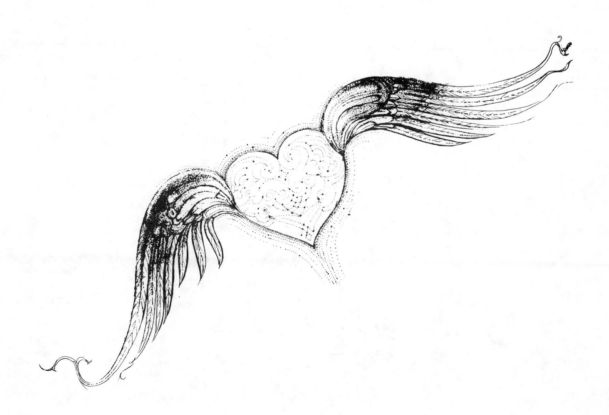